The

Environment

American Medical Association

of

Council on Long Range Planning and Development

Medicine

Contents

3

Health Care Resources

4

Changing Roles in the Health Sector

5

Conclusions and Implications

Established in 1970, the AMA Council on Long Range Planning and Development has several responsibilities, including the charge to identify and analyze trends in the environment of medicine. In fulfilling that charge, the Council has prepared a number of detailed environmental analysis reports over the years, including its most comprehensive report, *The Environment of Medicine (EOM)*. First published in 1983, the *EOM* was updated in 1984 and 1985.

This edition of the EOM is substantially different from previous editions of the report. In the past, the *EOM* discussed supply of and demand for health care resources and the factors affecting supply and demand. This latest edition of the report discusses more of the macrotrends affecting medicine: trends in the evolving health care economy, the growing supply of physicians, the changing demographic profile of the US population, and public and private sector initiatives affecting the practice of medicine. The report also discusses several major issues affecting health care: reimbursement of physicians, quality of care, professional liability, shortage of nurses, mandated health care plans, long-term care, and the acquired immunodeficiency syndrome (AIDS).

The future environment of medicine promises to be fast-paced and exciting. Despite some recent pronouncements by others to the contrary, the Council firmly believes that the future for medical practice is bright. New challenges will continue to confront physicians, but with these challenges will be unsurpassed opportunities for personal and professional gratification through dedicated service to patients and the community.

t is generally agreed that the United States has the best health care system in the world. Physicians in the United States have more resources at their disposal, have access to the latest technologic innovations, and have more autonomy than physicians in other countries. The fact that the United States remains the premier country in which to practice medicine is underscored by the influx of some of the world's best minds to practice medicine in the United States.

Under the leadership of physicians, the health status of the population has improved substantially. The incidence of many diseases common in the 1940s and 1950s, such as poliomyelitis, diptheria, and pertussis, has been reduced or eliminated. In addition, deaths from diseases such as ischemic heart disease, pneumonia, and tuberculosis have been reduced dramatically. Consequently, life expectancy at birth has increased from 54.1 years in 1920 to 74.7 years in 1985.

Despite the tremendous advances in medicine, US physicians are facing several challenges. Rapid advances in medical technology, although exciting, are placing constant pressure on physicians to remain knowledgeable in their field. Cost pressures continue to impinge upon established physicians' practice patterns. The increasingly litigious nature of the US society is impinging on the physician-patient relationship. Physicians are often frustrated by the difficulty in reaching medically underserved groups, such as adolescents and uninsured individuals.

While cost containment pressures, professional liability problems, and increasing federal government intervention are a few of the challenges confronting medicine, advances in disease prevention, new methods of diagnosis, and new treatment modalities are allowing US physicians to provide better, more effective care to their patients than ever before.

As Medicine prepares to meet these challenges, it will face the overarching issue of the nurture and protection of professionalism. This implies a strengthened commitment on the part of physicians to self-discipline and service to patients and to the public interest. Such a social contract will help assure independence in clinical decision-making and a strong physician-patient relationship. The Council on Long Range Planning and Development believes that these elements of professionalism constitute the basis for providing high quality medical care at reasonable cost, which is the shared goal of the American people and physicians.

This report studies four major areas of the environment of medicine:

☐ The Economics of the Health Care Sector;

☐ Demographic Trends;

☐ Health Care Resources; and

☐ Roles of the Key Participants in Health Care and the Key Issues to be Addressed.

In 1988, the US economy entered the seventh year of its longest peacetime expansion in history: the economy grew at a rate above its expected long-term growth rate; the unemployment rate in 1988 fell to its lowest level since the mid-1970s; and price inflation remained under control.

The health care sector created 11 percent of the goods and services produced in the United States in 1987. Between 1980 and 1987, national expenditures for health care grew rapidly. The components of the health sector expenditures growing the fastest include:

☐ Other Professional Services;

☐ Program Administration; and

☐ Physician Services.

The rapidly growing health care economy continues to place financial pressure on those who pay for health care services. Consequently, payors will continue to implement programs to contain their health care costs. Cost containment programs in the past have focused primarily on hospital expenditures, but they are likely to focus increasingly on physician expenditures. As cost containment measures continue to alter the practice of medicine, concerns over their effects on the quality of medical care will grow.

Despite the implementation of many cost containment programs, the Health Care Financing Administration (HCFA) projects that, by the year 2000, the health care sector will produce $1.5 trillion in US goods and services, which will represent an estimated 15 percent of total US output in that year.

The HCFA projection assumes that the US economy will continue to grow moderately with low inflation. There are, however, several potential economic issues that may affect those assumptions, including a rising rate of inflation, problems with the solvency of savings and loan associations, and the growing federal debt. Each of these factors has the potential to precipitate an economic downturn in the United States, with an impact on the health care sector.

Demographic
Characteristics
of the US
Population

The growth of the US population will continue to exert upward pressure on the demand for physician services, but at a slowing pace. While increasing by over 18 percent in the 1950s, the US population grew by only 11 percent in the 1970s. The US Census Bureau projects that the US population is likely to grow by around 7 percent during the 1990s and by less than 6 percent between 2000-2010.

Concomitant with the slowing growth of the US population is the aging of the population. Between 1988 and 2025, the US population is projected to increase by only 23 percent, but the 45-59 age group is expected to increase by 52 percent; the 60-74 age bracket is projected to increase by over 85 percent; and the 75 and over age group is estimated to grow by over 98 percent. Consequently, the demand for the services of physicians who treat older citizens can be expected to increase (holding other factors constant). In contrast, the demand for the services of physicians who treat younger individuals is not expected to rise as fast because of the projected decline in the 15-29 year age group and the projected slow growth of the 0-14 age group.

Based on historical trends, the specialties projected to grow the fastest between 1985 and 2000 are:

☐ Emergency Medicine;

☐ All medical subspecialties as a group; and

☐ Anesthesiology.

The specialties projected to grow the slowest are:

☐ General Surgery;

☐ Pathology; and

☐ General/Family Practice.

The growth in the supply of physicians is projected to exceed the growth in the US population between 1985 and 2000. In addition, the AMA estimates that the growth in the supply of physicians will exceed the growth in the utilization of physicians' services by about 10 percent between 1985 and 2000. However, the specialties of general/family practice, general surgery, and psychiatry are projected to grow at a slower rate than the growth in the utilization of their services.

It is widely acknowledged that there is a shortage of nurses in the United States. Only 17.6 percent of hospitals surveyed reported having no RN vacancies in 1986-1987. This shortage situation appears likely to continue for several years and may contribute to a further restructuring of the health care delivery system.

The delivery of health care will continue to shift away from hospital-based care. Between 1976 and 1986, the number of community hospitals declined by 3.1 percent, while the number of ambulatory surgical centers and health maintenance organizations has been growing. Between 1984 and 1988, Independent Practice Association (IPA) HMOs have emerged as the dominant form of HMO. There have been signs, however, of a leveling off in the growth of HMOs.

The roles of the key participants in the health care sector are
continuing to evolve. The federal government is attempting to shift its
role from "price-taker" to "price-maker." It is expected that the financial
outlay of the federal government to health care will continue to grow.
Cost containment in health care will continue to be a major goal of the
federal government.

US businesses assumed a largely passive role in the health system
until the 1970s. However, as the US economy has turned into a global
economy, US businesses have become much more careful about
expenditures which make them less competitive in the global market.
Health care costs are major expenses for many companies and, as a
result, businesses can be expected to continue to adopt a more activist
role in containing health care costs.

Organized labor remains committed to preserving the health benefits
currently in place and is pressing for health insurance coverage for the
many employees who are currently uninsured.

In the past, insurers acted as a "pass through" mechanism for health
expenditures. However, the health care insurance sector has become
increasingly competitive over the past several years. To maintain
positive financial results, health insurers are exploring new methods to
accurately anticipate utilization and to control payouts.

Patients are becoming increasingly aware of personal health issues.
Public opinion polls show that US citizens are more concerned with
what they eat and drink and are more aware of the relationships between
healthful lifestyles and overall health status. Consequently, the general
public is becoming more active in the health care decision-making
process.

Economic pressures are the driving force behind the changing
structure of the hospital sector. As pressures to contain charges have
increased and the federal government has imposed more and more constraints on Medicare and Medicaid reimbursement, the hospital sector

has undergone structural change in order to increase efficiency and diversify the sources of hospital revenues.

Organized medicine is actively addressing a number of critical issues affecting physicians, including professional liability, quality of care, and Medicare and Medicaid reform. These and many other issues will continue to be addressed by organized medicine in the coming years.

Some of the major issues that are expected to develop considerable discussion among these key participants in the health care sector in 1989 and later years include the following:

☐ Reimbursement of Physicians

☐ Quality of Care Evaluation and Assurance

☐ Professional Liability

☐ Shortage of Nurses

☐ Health Expense Protection for the Uninsured

☐ Long-Term Care

☐ Acquired Immunodeficiency Syndrome (AIDS).

There are several conclusions that can be drawn from the latest trends affecting medicine, including:

Conclusions and
Implications

Theme 1. Cost pressures will continue to be the principal driving force underlying change in the medical care environment.

Theme 2. As cost containment pressures continue to grow, pressures will mount to develop effective methods for evaluating and assuring the quality of health care.

Theme 3. Advances in medical technology will continue to strongly influence change in the environment of medicine.

Theme 4. Fundamental shifts in the demographic characteristics of the US population will have a major effect on the long range demand for medical care services.

Theme 5. The supply of physicians is projected to increase at a faster rate than the US population overall.

Theme 6. Governmental initiatives are likely to continue to be a major source of change in the environment of medicine.

Theme 7. Health policy issues will become increasingly pollticized.

Theme 8. Changes in the environment of medicine may lead to unexpected divisions and alliances on health policy issues.

Theme 9. The environment of the health care sector will become more uncertain.

Many of the trends contained in this report suggest that the environment of medicine is likely to undergo further evolution in the near future. It appears that this evolution, if it occurs, will involve a continuing restructuring of the medical care financing and delivery systems. But, given the uncertainties about the magnitude and direction of several key environmental trends, the development of a specific forecast of the future environment of medicine is very difficult. Therefore, the AMA's Council on Long Range Planning and Development has not attempted to make a specific prediction on the mechanisms through which medical care will be financed and delivered in the future, except to suggest that change is likely. The Council has, however, attempted to provide background information and interpretations of that information as the basis upon which the reader can develop his or her own perspectives and conclusions on the future environment of medicine.

Two factors should be balanced against the view that further evolution in the environment of medicine is likely in the near future:

1. There is an inherent tendency in undertaking a study of the environment to search for and emphasize the forces for change. The reader should keep in mind that there are strong forces that will resist radical changes in the environment of medicine. Both the public and physicians express strong support for almost all aspects of the current medical care system, except for the "costs" of that system. All the major participants in the health sector consistently express satisfaction and pride in the

quality of medical care in this country.

2. There is less than complete certainty about the ramifications of many of the environmental trends identified and analyzed in this report. There is even less certainty about how various environmental trends are likely to interact with each other. It is possible that some environmental trends may completely offset others. Again, the reader is encouraged to embrace healthy skepticism about accepting the view that rapid change in the environment of medicine is inevitable. History demonstrates that individuals and systems usually prove to be more resilient than expected.

1

The Economics of
the Health Sector
Economy

n 1988, the US economy entered the seventh year of the longest peacetime expansion in its history. Economic growth was strong, with the economy's real output growing by around 4 percent in 1988. Prices increased moderately, moving up by about 4 percent as measured by the consumer price index. Employment grew, with less than 6 percent of the labor force unemployed. Judged in comparison with the economic climate of the prior 8 years, the US economy enjoyed a good year in 1988 (see Figure 1.1).

Figure 1.1

Change in Real
Gross National
Product, Consumer
Prices, and
Unemployment

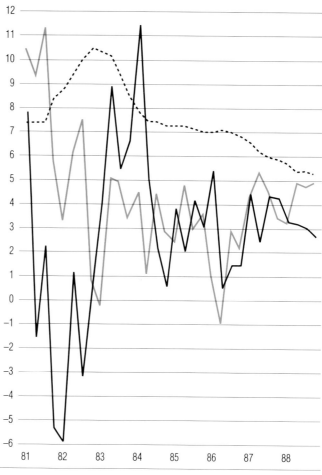

—— Gross National
    Product

—— Inflation Rate

---- Unemployment

Sources: Economic Report of the President, selected issues. *Survey of Current Business*, selected issues. 1986 data from *Blue Chip Economic Indicators*, September 10, 1988.

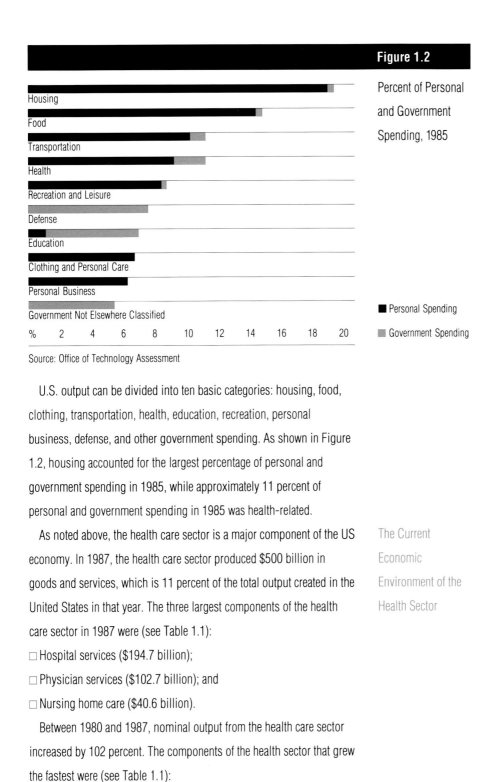

Figure 1.2

Percent of Personal
and Government
Spending, 1985

Housing

Food

Transportation

Health

Recreation and Leisure

Defense

Education

Clothing and Personal Care

Personal Business

Government Not Elsewhere Classified

% 2 4 6 8 10 12 14 16 18 20

■ Personal Spending

■ Government Spending

Source: Office of Technology Assessment

U.S. output can be divided into ten basic categories: housing, food, clothing, transportation, health, education, recreation, personal business, defense, and other government spending. As shown in Figure 1.2, housing accounted for the largest percentage of personal and government spending in 1985, while approximately 11 percent of personal and government spending in 1985 was health-related.

As noted above, the health care sector is a major component of the US economy. In 1987, the health care sector produced $500 billion in goods and services, which is 11 percent of the total output created in the United States in that year. The three largest components of the health care sector in 1987 were (see Table 1.1):

☐ Hospital services ($194.7 billion);

☐ Physician services ($102.7 billion); and

☐ Nursing home care ($40.6 billion).

Between 1980 and 1987, nominal output from the health care sector increased by 102 percent. The components of the health sector that grew the fastest were (see Table 1.1):

Table 1.1

National Health
Expenditures, 1987

Type of Expenditure	Amount in Billions 1987	Percentage Change 1980-87
National Health Expenditures	$ 500.3	102%
Health Services and Supplies	483.2	105
Personal Health Care	442.6	101
Hospital Care	194.7	92
Physician Services	102.7	119
Dentist Services	32.8	113
Other Professional Services	16.2	184
Nondurable Medical Products	34.0	81
Durable Medical Products	9.5	86
Nursing Home Care	40.6	99
Other Personal Health Care	12.0	103
Program Administration and Net Cost of Private Health Insurance	25.9	182
Government Public Health Activities	14.7	101
Research and Construction	17.1	44

Source: U.S. Department of Health and Human Services.

☐ *Other professional services*, which reflects the costs of services of nonphysician professionals such as optometrists and podiatrists;

☐ *Program administration and net cost of private health insurance*, which includes operating expenses of private health insurance organizations; and

☐ *Physician services*, which reflects the costs of services provided by physicians.

There are three basic sources of financing for health care. As indicated in Table 1.2, about 25 percent of the cost of health care is paid directly by the patient, almost 32 percent is paid for through private insurance

Table 1.2

	Percentage of National Health Care Expenditures*	National Health Care Expenditures	National Health Care Expenditures by Source of Funds, 1987
All Sources	$500.3	100%	
Private Funds	293.0	59	
Direct from Patient	123.0	25	
Private Insurance	157.8	32	
Philanthropy	12.2	2	
Public Funds	207.3	41	
Federal Government	144.7	29	
State and Local Governments	62.7	12	

Source: U.S. Department of Health and Human Services. *Amount in billions.

(Numbers may not add due to rounding.)

companies, and slightly over 41 percent is paid by local, state, and federal governments. The largest single purchaser of health care in the United States is the federal government.

Examining the budget of the federal government, however, indicates that health care expenditures are only a fraction of the federal government's total budget. *In 1987, health and medicare comprised 11 percent of the total federal budget, while national defense comprised 28 percent of the budget, social security comprised 21 percent, and interest payments comprised 14 percent.* In addition, between 1980 and 1987, national defense grew by 110 percent, interest payments increased by 185 percent, and health and medicare rose by 109 percent.

International comparisons are frequently made with respect to national health care expenditures. Figure 1.3 indicates the percentage of gross domestic product (GDP) devoted to health care for several countries. In 1986, the share of health expenditures in GDP was 11 percent in the United States, 9.1 percent in Sweden, and 3.6 percent in Turkey. Canada

International Comparisons

Table 1.3

Federal Budget,
1980 and 1987

	1980 Actual Outlays	Percent of Total	1987 Actual Outlays	Percent of Total
National Defense	$134	23%	$282	28%
Health and Medicare	55	9	115	11
Income Security	87	15	123	12
Social Security	119	20	207	21
Interest Payments	53	9	139	14
Other	143	24	139	14
Total	$591	100%	$1,005	100%

Source: *Economic Report of the President,* February 1988, Table B-77.

*Amount in billions.

expended about 8.5 percent of its GDP for health care. Thus, compared with other countries, the US spends a relatively higher proportion of its annual production on health care.

There are many shortcomings in international comparisons of health expenditures, however. For example, some countries have older populations with greater health care needs, causing their health care expenditures to rise. Access to care, generally, and to new medical procedures and technologies, specifically, can result in significant differences in health expenditures between various countries. Countries also define and classify health care expenditures differently, such as spending for school and prison health services. And, some countries are wealthier than others, which accounts for some spending differences. Consequently, caution should be used in comparing health care data between countries.

Outlook for the
Future of the
Health Care Sector

Assuming the US economy continues to grow moderately, as it did in 1988, the Health Care Financing Administration (HCFA) is projecting that the health sector will produce $1.5 trillion of goods and services by the year 2000 which represents an estimated 15 percent of all US output

Figure 1.3

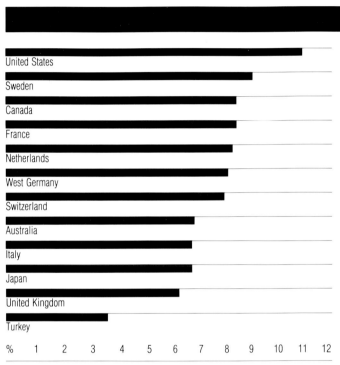

United States	
Sweden	
Canada	
France	
Netherlands	
West Germany	
Switzerland	
Australia	
Italy	
Japan	
United Kingdom	
Turkey	

% 1 2 3 4 5 6 7 8 9 10 11 12

Health Expenditures as a Percentage of Gross Domestic Product, 1986

Source: Fall 1988, *Health Affairs*

Table 1.4

Health Care Expenditures

Year	Gross National Product (Amount in Billions)	National Health Care Expenditures	Percent of GNP
1980	$2,732	$248.1	9.1%
1984	3,765	391.1	10.4
1985	3,998	422.6	10.6
1986	4,206	458.2	10.9
1987 (Projected)	4,433	496.6	11.2
1990 (Projected)	5,414	647.3	12.0
1995 (Projected)	7,467	999.1	13.4
2000 (Projected)	10,164	1,529.3	15.0

Source: National Health Expenditures, 1986-2000. *Health Care Financing Review*,

1987;8:1-36.

Table 1.5

National Health
Expenditures*,
1986-2000

	2000	1986	Percent Change
National Health Expenditures	1,529.3	458.2	234
Health services and supplies	1,493.8	442.0	238
Personal health care	1,398.1	404.0	246
Hospital care	621.0	179.6	246
Physician services	319.6	92.0	247
Dentist services	89.6	29.6	203
Other professional services	60.4	14.1	328
Drugs and medical sundries	102.6	30.6	235
Eyeglasses and appliances	24.7	8.2	201
Nursing home care	129.0	38.1	239
Other personal health care	51.2	11.9	330
Program administration and net cost of private health insurance	57.7	24.5	136
Government public health activities	38.0	13.4	184
Research and construction of medical facilities	35.5	16.3	118

Source: National Health Expenditures, 1986-2000. *Health Care Financing Review*, 1987;8:1-36. *Amount in billions.

in that year (see Table 1.4). These projections indicate that the health care sector will become an even more important factor in the US economy in the future.

Table 1.5 presents detailed HCFA projections on the growth in health care expenditures between 1986 and 2000. The expenditure categories projected to grow the fastest are:

☐ Other personal health care (330%),

☐ Other professional services (328%), and

☐ Physician services (247%).

Interestingly, the HCFA projections suggest that the costs of program administration, one of the three components of the health care sector

	National Health Care Expenditures For Physician Care*	Proportion Paid by Patients	Proportion Paid by Private Health Insurance	Proportion Paid By Government	National Expenditures for Physician Care
1980	$46.8	30.3%	42.7%	26.9%	
1985	82.8	27.8	42.9	29.2	
1986	92.0	28.5	42.1	29.4	
1987	102.7	27.8	41.9	30.3	
1990	132.6	26.5	41.3	32.2	
1995	209.0	23.8	40.2	35.9	
2000	319.6	23.7	39.7	36.6	

Source: National Health Expenditures, 1986-2000, *Health Care Financing Review*, 1987;8:1-36. *Amount in billions.

growing the fastest between 1980 and 1987, will increase at a slower rate in the future.

Outlook for Physicians' Services. As indicated in Table 1.6, HCFA projects that expenditures for physicians' services will increase from $101.4 billion in 1987 to $319.6 billion in the year 2000, an increase of 215 percent.

As the physician service component of the health sector grows, the proportion of physician care expenditures paid by federal, state and local governments is projected to rise. As indicated in Table 1.6, HCFA projects that the proportion of physician care expenditures paid by all levels of government will increase from 30 percent in 1987 to almost 37 percent in the year 2000. Conversely, the amount of physician care paid by patients and by private third-party payors is projected to decline through 2000. If governments increase their funding for physician services, as projected, it can be expected that they will continue to attempt to exert a growing influence on the practice of medicine.

Table 1.7

National

Expenditures for

Hospital Care

Year	National Expenditures for Hospital Care*	Proportion Paid By Patients	Proportion Paid By Private Health Insurance	Proportion Paid By Government	Proportion Paid By Other Private Financing
1980	$101.6	7.8%	38.1%	53.1%	1.1%
1985	167.2	8.7	36.2	53.9	1.2
1986	179.6	9.4	36.1	53.3	1.2
1987	194.7	10.6	37.3	50.8	1.2
1990	250.4	9.8	36.5	52.5	1.2
1995	393.6	10.9	35.4	52.4	1.2
2000	621.0	12.0	34.4	52.4	1.2

Source: National Health Expenditures, 1986-2000, *Health Care Financing Review*, Summer 1987. *Amount in billions.

Outlook for Hospital Care. Between 1987 and 2000, HCFA projects that the value of hospital services will increase from $192.6 billion to $621.0 billion, an increase of 223 percent.

While patients are expected to pay for a declining proportion of their physician care, they are projected to pay for a rising proportion of their hospital care. As indicated in Table 1.7, the proportion of hospital care paid by patients has risen from 7.8 percent in 1980 to 10.6 percent in 1987. By the year 2000, it is projected that about 12 percent of hospital costs will be paid for directly by patients through higher deductibles and higher co-insurance. Thus, patients can be expected to become more sensitive to the cost of hospital services in the future, as they pay for a greater proportion of their hospital care.

Economic Concerns. The projections above assume continued growth in the US economy, with moderate inflation. There are, however, several potential factors that may affect these assumptions.

Growing Rate of Price Inflation. Over the past several years, the Federal Reserve Board has been playing a greater role in the US economy. The Federal Reserve Board's primary concern is the rate of inflation in the US economy. If the rate of inflation begins to increase, it is likely that the Federal Reserve Board will move to raise interest rates. Higher interest rates tend to reduce price inflation, but they also tend to reduce economic growth. If inflation surges, it could be expected that the Federal Reserve Board would act to raise interest rates and, thereby, slow economic growth.

The Savings and Loan Problems. As the banking industry was de-regulated, much of the preferential status and regulatory oversight of savings and loan associations was reduced or eliminated. As a result, many savings and loan associations are on the brink of financial disaster. About one-third of the savings and loan associations are unprofitable. Estimates project a cost of about $100 billion to return the savings and loan associations to solvency. The impact of this problem on the US economy and on the health care sector will depend on how it is handled at the state and federal government levels.

The Federal Debt. From 1980 to 1988, the debt of the Federal government grew rapidly. As indicated in Figure 1.4, federal expenditures have outpaced federal revenues during the l980s, causing the federal debt to rise considerably. It is expected that the federal government will become increasingly restrictive in its expenditures in the future. Programs receiving federal funds should expect continued attempts at budgetary restrictions.

Figure 1.4

Total Federal Debt
(in trillions)

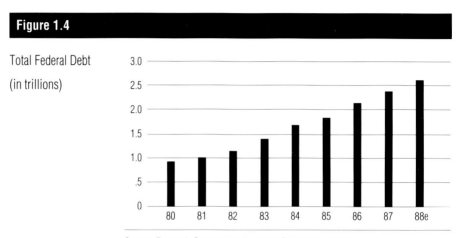

Source: *Economic Report of the President*, February 1988, Table B-77.

2

Demographic Trends

The US health care system is considered by most to be the best in the world. It is also, however, considered one of the most expensive systems in the world. In 1986, approximately 11 percent of the US gross national product went to expenditures for health care. One trend contributing to the rising cost of health care is the growth of and changes in the US population.

After discussing the projected growth in the demand for health care services between 1985 and 2000, this section discusses the demographic forces and trends that are affecting the US health care system, such as:

1. Population Growth Rate
2. Age Distribution
3. Sex Composition
4. Racial Composition
5. Migration Patterns
6. Health Status
7. AIDS

Projected Growth in the Utilization of Physician Services

In 1988, the AMA Center for Health Policy Research completed a comprehensive study of the future utilization of physician services, based on current utilization rates. As indicated in Table 2.1, the study concludes that the future utilization of physician services is likely to increase by around 14 percent between 1985 and 2000 (barring any unforeseen changes in prices, incomes, epidemiology or other factors that would significantly affect utilization rates). In addition, the study shows that the number of physician contacts will increase for each major specialty, from a low of 3 percent in obstetrics and gynecology to a high of almost 25 percent in general internal medicine. The next several sections of this chapter provide a discussion of the demographic factors affecting the growth in the utilization of physician services in the future.

Population Growth Rate

Census studies have shown that the growth of the US population has been slowing. After increasing by almost 19 percent in the 1950s, the US

Table 2.1

	Growth Rate in Total Contacts, 1985-2000	
All Physicians	14.55%	Projected Growth in Patient Contacts by Specialty, 1985-2000
General/Family Practice	13.03	
General Internal Medicine	24.56	
Medical Subspecialties	23.43	
General Surgery	16.50	
Surgical Subspecialties	17.14	
Pediatrics	6.98	
Obstetrics/Gynecology	2.83	
Psychiatry	19.42	
Emergency Medicine	6.20	

Source: AMA Center for Health Policy Research, 1988.

population increased by slightly less than 14 percent during the 1960s and by only 11 percent during the 1970s. The US Bureau of the Census projects that the slowing growth rate of the US population is likely to continue. The Bureau predicts that the population will increase by 9.6 percent during the 1980s, by 7.3 percent during the 1990s, and by 5.7 percent during the first decade of the next century. This information is depicted in Figure 2.1.

Surveys conducted during the 1970s and 1980s indicate that the number of physician visits per person have averaged between 4.6 and 5.1 visits per year. If physician visits per person remain in this range, the slowing growth rate of the population may be one factor tending to restrain growth in the demand for physician services in the future, thereby acting to reduce the upward pressure on health care expenditures. However, this must be viewed in light of projected changes in the age distribution of the US population.

Projections from the US Bureau of the Census indicate that the age

Age Distribution

Figure 2.1

Population Trends
and Projections
(in millions)

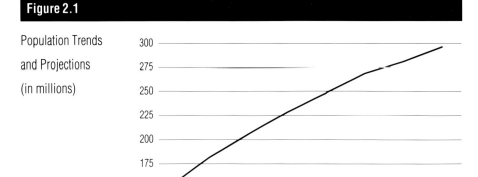

Source: Statistical Abstract of the United States 1987, Tables 2 and 14, and Bureau of the Census: *Projections of the Population of the United States, by Age, Sex, and Race: 1983 to 2080.* Series P-25, No. 952.

distribution of the US population will change considerably between now and the year 2000. As indicated in Table 2.2, the US population is projected to increase by 9.2 percent between 1988 and 2000. The age groups growing the fastest during this period are likely to be the 45-59 age group and the 75 and older age group. The 15-29 year age group is projected to experience a 10 percent decline in numbers, and the 60-74 year age bracket is likely to experience a 1 percent fall in numbers. However, between 1988 and 2025, all of the older age brackets are projected to experience considerable increases in numbers, while the younger age groups are projected to grow little, if at all.

Utilization of health care services, in general, and physician services, in particular, has been shown to be directly related to the age distribution of the population. In a recent study of consumer behavior, the utilization rate of physician services was estimated. As illustrated in Table 2.3, children under age 17 see physicians slightly over 3 times per year on average. Adults, 75 years and older, however, see physicians approximately 11 times a year on average. Holding other factors constant, the utilization of physician services is likely to increase as the US population ages.

Table 2.2

	In Thousands			Percentage Change		Age Distribution of
Age Group	1988	2000	2025	1988-2000	1988-2025	the US Population,
0–14	53,156	55,903	55,235	5.2%	3.9%	1988-2025
15–29	59,360	53,484	55,178	−9.9	−7.0	
30–44	56,707	62,762	59,735	10.7	5.3	
45–59	34,740	50,399	52,927	45.1	52.4	
60–74	28,439	28,164	52,735	−1.0	85.4	
75+	12,902	17,244	25,583	33.7	98.3	
Total	245,302	267,955	301,394	9.2	22.9	

Source: US Bureau of the Census: *Projections of the Population of the United States by Age, Sex, and Race: 1983-2080*, table 2, middle series.

Table 2.3

Age	Visits/year	Estimated Per
Under 17	3.2	Person Physician
17-24	3.6	Visits Per Year
25-44	4.2	by Age
45-64	5.4	
65-74	8.1	
75+	10.9	

Source: WD Marder, PR Kletke, AB Silberger, RJ Willke: *Physician Supply and Utilization by Specialty: Trends and Projections,* February 1988.

Since older people utilize health care services at a higher rate than younger people, their expenditures are also higher. As indicated in Table 2.4, a consumer expenditure survey by the US Bureau of Labor Statistics found that individuals under age 25 spent an average of $305 out of pocket for health care in 1984, while individuals 75 years and over spent an average of $1,487 out of pocket. The study also indicated that the elderly devoted a higher percentage of their total yearly expenditures to

Table 2.4

Average Individual
Expenditures for
Health Care, 1984

Age Group	Amount	Health Expenditures as a Percent of Total Yearly Expenditures
Under 25	$305	2.3
25-34	626	2.9
35-44	795	2.9
45-54	1,061	3.7
55-64	1,060	4.6
65-74	1,340	8.4
75+	1,487	13.3

Source: US Department of Commerce: *Statistical Abstract of the United States, 1987,*
table 135.

health care in 1984 than did younger people.

One reason for the higher utilization of health care resources by the
elderly is the type of illnesses most prevalent among this population.
According to data published by the National Center for Health Statistics,
the population 65 years of age and older have a much lower incidence of
acute conditions than the population under 65 years of age. However, a
very large portion of the elderly suffer from chronic conditions such as
arteriosclerosis, senility, cerebrovascular disease, and mental disorders.
As the population ages, it is expected that the prevalence of chronic
disorders, and the costs associated therewith, will increase.

The utilization of physician services among the elderly varies by
physician specialty. A recent AMA study shows that the percent of
revenues from Medicare among physicians with any Medicare revenues
was highest for:

☐ Internal Medicine (40.2%);

☐ Pathology (33.9%);

☐ Radiology (33.2%); and

Table 2.5

	Female	Male	
Physician Visits	5.8	4.5	Comparison of
Dental Visits	2.0*	1.7*	Health Care
Discharges from Short-Stay Hospitals (per 1,000 population)	103.2	107.0	Utilization by Sex,
Days of Care in a Short-Stay Hospital (per 1,000 population)	703.8	793.3	1985
Average Length of Stay in a Short-Stay Hospital	6.8	7.4	

Source: US Department of Health and Human Services: *Health United States 1986 and Prevention Profile*, various tables. *1983 data.

□ Surgery (31.7%).

Thus, holding other factors constant, the increasing age of the US population could be expected to increase the demand, in particular, for these specialists.

Females tend to utilize more non-hospital health care services than do males. Data from the National Center for Health Statistics indicate that females have more physician and dental visits than males. However, males tend to utilize more hospital services than females, as indicated in Table 2.5.

Sex Composition

The proportion of female patients also varies across specialty groups. Females constitute a high proportion of the patients of obstetricians/ gynecologists, general/family practitioners, and internists.

Between 1985 and 2000, the projected utilization of physician services indicates a greater use of physician services by both genders, with a slightly greater increase in utilization of physician services by males than females. This is depicted in Table 2.6.

Projections indicate that the non-white population is likely to grow approximately three times faster than the white population between 1980 and 2000 (see Table 2.7). While the white population is projected to increase by about 9 percent between 1980 and 2000, the non-white

Racial Composition

Table 2.6

Projected Utilization of Physician Services per 1,000 Population by Sex	1985	2000	1985-2000 Percent Change
Total Physician Contacts	4,664.9	4,785.6	2.6%
Male	3,623.7	3,725.3	2.8
Female	5,635.0	5,780.3	2.6

Source: WD Marder, PR Kletke, AB Silberger, RJ Willke: *Physician Supply and Utilization by Specialty: Trends and Projections,* February 1988.

population is expected to grow by almost 27 percent during the period.

The US Census Bureau reported that the Hispanic population is growing at a rate almost five times faster than the rest of the US population. More than half of all Hispanics live in California (33.9%) or Texas (21.3%). In 1988, there were about 19.4 million Americans of Hispanic descent.

The utilization of health services varies by race. In 1985, utilization of physicians per capita was 14 percent higher for whites than non-whites. As the racial composition of the U.S. population changes, physicians are likely to see a higher proportion of non-whites in their patient population.

Besides differences in utilization rates, racial composition also affects the types of health conditions seen by physicians. Figure 2.2 indicates that whites have a higher rate of infective conditions but a lower rate of digestive problems than either blacks or hispanics.

Blacks are more likely to experience digestive problems but less likely to have respiratory problems than whites or hispanics.

Migration

The US population in general is mobile. For several economic and social reasons, the US population has been migrating South and West. This situation suggests that many of the rapidly growing areas of the nation will experience increasing demand for physicians' services. At the same time, other areas may experience a decline in the demand for

Table 2.7

	1980 Population	1980-2000	
	In Thousands	Percent Change	Projected
Total	222,218	11.7%	Population Growth
Race			Rates By Race,
White	191,164	9.0%	1980-2000
Non-white	31,054	27.1%	

Source: Marder WD, et al: *Physician Supply and Utilization by Specialty: Trends and Projections.* Chicago, American Medical Association, 1988, Table 7.1.

Figure 2.2

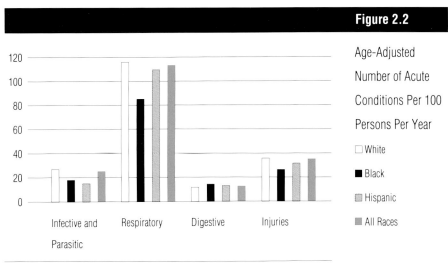

Age-Adjusted Number of Acute Conditions Per 100 Persons Per Year

☐ White
■ Black
▦ Hispanic
▨ All Races

Source: Health Indicators for Hispanic, Black, and White Americans. *Vital and Health Statistics,* Series 10, No. 148, September 1984.

physicians' services.

Table 2.8 indicates that the population is projected to grow rapidly in the South and West. The Northeast and Midwest regions are projected to have a negative population growth rate during the 1990s. Thus, the future growth in the utilization of physician services is likely to vary considerably by region of the country.

The health status of the US population has been improving, as indicated by various measures. One measure of the health status of the

Health Status

Table 2.8

Population Trends
and Projections by
Region of the
Country

	Percentage Change During Decade			
	Northeast	Midwest	South	West
1950	13.2%	16.0%	16.5%	39.1%
1960	9.8	9.7	14.2	23.8
1970	0.0	4.1	20.1	24.1
1980	−1.4	2.4	16.2	22.5
1990	−4.1	−1.0	12.8	18.1

Source: *Statistical Abstract of the United States 1987.* Table 23.

nation is the infant mortality rate. In 1960, the number of infant deaths in the US averaged 26.0 per 1,000 live births. By 1985, the rate had fallen to 10.6 deaths per 1,000 live births. Another measure of the health status of the nation is the age-adjusted death rates. In 1950, there were 841.5 deaths per 100,000 resident population. By 1985, that rate had fallen to 545.9 deaths per 100,000 resident population. As indicated in Table 2.9, the incidence rate of some notifiable diseases has been declining, while the incidence of others has been increasing. For example, the number of cases of diphtheria has fallen from 5,800 cases in 1950 to 1 case in 1984, while gonorrhea has increased from 287,000 cases in 1950 to 878,000 cases in 1984. It is likely that physicians will continue to see a shift in the types of cases they treat.

Acquired Immune
Deficiency
Syndrome

The first cases of the Acquired Immune Deficiency Syndrome (AIDS) were reported to the Centers for Disease Control (CDC) in 1981. Since that time the incidence of and associated mortality from AIDS in the United States has increased inexorably. As indicated in Figure 2.3, the number of diagnosed cases of AIDS increased from 271 cases in 1981 and prior years to 20,159 in 1987. Deaths from AIDS rose from 250 in 1981 and prior years to 9,299 in 1986, falling slightly in 1987 to 6,655. The CDC projects that the number of new cases of AIDS per year will likely rise from about 33,000 in 1988 to about 74,000 in 1991, an

Disease	1950	1960	1970	1980	1984
AIDS	—	—	—	—	4,445
Diphtheria	5,796	918	435	3	1
Hepatitis A	—	41,666	56,797	29,087	22,040
Hepatitis B	—		8,310	19,015	26,115
Mumps	—	—	104,953	8,576	3,021
Pertussis (whooping cough)	120,718	14,809	4,249	1,730	2,276
Poliomyelitis, total	33,300	3,190	33	9	8
Paralytic		2,525	31	8	8
Rubella (German measles)	—	—	56,552	3,904	752
Rubeola (measles)	319,124	441,703	47,351	13,506	2,587
Salmonellosis, excluding typhoid fever	—	6,929	22,096	33,715	40,861
Shigellosis	23,367	12,487	13,845	19,041	17,371
Tuberculosis	121,742	55,494	37,137	27,749	22,255
Varicella (chickenpox)	—	—	—	190,894	221,983
Sexually transmitted diseases					
Syphilis, total	217,558	122,538	91,382	68,832	69,888
Primary and secondary	23,939	16,145	21,982	27,204	28,607
Early latent	59,256	18,017	16,311	20,297	23,132
Late and late latent	113,569	81,798	50,348	20,979	17,827
Congenital	13,377	4,416	1,953	277	322
Gonorrhea	286,746	258,933	600,072	1,004,029	878,556
Chancroid	4,977	1,680	1,416	788	665
Granuloma inguinale	1,783	296	124	51	30
Lymphogranuloma venereum	1,427	835	612	199	170

Source: US Department of Health and Human Services: Health United States 1986 and Prevention Profile, various tables.

Table 2.9

The Number of Cases of Selected Notifiable Diseases

Figure 2.3

Incidence and
Associated
Mortality of AIDS in
the United States
(in thousands)

—— Number of
    Diagnosed Cases
– – Projected
—— Number of Deaths
– – Projected

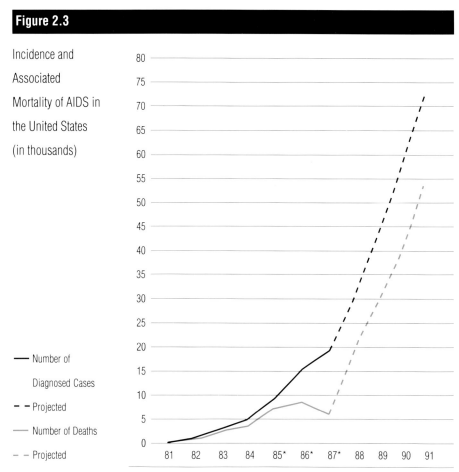

Sources: Morgan WM, Curran JW: Acquired Immunodeficiency Syndrome: Current and

Future Trends, *Public Health Reports*, September-October 1986, 101:5, 459-465.

*CDC Weekly Surveillance Reports, AMA/NET AIDS Information Service, April 8, 1988.

increase of 124 percent. Deaths are also projected to increase from
about 21,000 in 1988 to about 54,000 in 1991.

The age distribution of AIDS patients is centered around the 30-39
age bracket. About 46 percent of the AIDS patients at the time of diagnosis were between the ages of 30 and 39. An additional 21 percent of
the patients were between the ages of 20 and 29, and a similar percentage of patients were between the ages of 40 and 49. Overall, nine of ten
AIDS patients were between ages 20-49 at the time of AIDS diagnosis.

The geographic distribution of patients with AIDS is uneven across the United States. Of the cumulative number of cases of AIDS, about 26 percent were in New York State, 22 percent were in California, and between five and ten percent were in each of three states: Florida, New Jersey, and Texas.

Several studies have estimated the cost of medical care for AIDS treatment. Early reports suggested that hospital charges for patients with AIDS may be as high as $147,000 per patient. Subsequent reports, however, indicate that the costs may be significantly lower.

Recently, two separate reports have placed the cost of treating the AIDS victim in the $60,000 to $80,000 range. Assuming that this estimate is accurate, the lifetime cost of treating the 15,864 AIDS cases diagnosed in 1986 would be in the range of $952 million — $1.3 billion. If the CDC projections are accurate, the cost of treating the 74,000 cases of AIDS diagnosed in 1991 would be approximately $4.4 billion — $5.9 billion. In comparison, the U.S. national health expenditures in the United States were an estimated $497 billion in 1987.

Table 2.10 helps put AIDS in perspective with other causes of death. In 1986, nearly half of the deaths in the United States were caused by cardiovascular diseases, while pneumonia and influenza caused 70,500 deaths in that year. AIDS in 1986 contributed to 9,299 deaths. Thus, AIDS is not a leading cause of death at this time. However, the number of deaths from AIDS is growing rapidly. If the projected number of deaths from AIDS in 1991 had occurred in 1986, AIDS would have been about the seventh leading cause of death in that year.

Table 2.10

Ten Leading Causes
of Death in the
United States, 1986

	Deaths
Total Deaths	2,099,000
Major Cardiovascular Diseases	967,930
Malignancies	465,980
Accidents	95,640
Chronic Obstructive Pulmonary Disease	75,420
Pneumonia and Influenza	70,500
Diabetes Mellitus	36,340
Suicide	31,470
Chronic Liver Disease and Cirrhosis	26,210
Nephritis, Nephrotic Syndrome, and Nephrosis	21,790
Homicide and Legal Intervention	21,400

Source: Monthly Vital Statistics Report, August 1987.

3

Health Care
Resources

The supply of health care resources has been growing rapidly in recent years, but the demand for those resources has also been growing. Consequently, the health sector has been able to absorb, for the most part, the increasing supply of health care resources. Questions have arisen recently about the capacity of the sector to continue to absorb rapid increases in resources. If the supply of health care resources continues to grow rapidly while growth in demand slows, pressures will develop which are likely to cause further changes in the environment of medicine.

This chapter reviews recent and projected trends in the supply of physicians, nurses, allied health personnel, and the delivery of physician services.

Recent Trends in Physician Manpower

From 1970 to 1986, the number of active U.S. physicians increased from 311,203 to 519,411, a 67 percent increase.* This increase indicates that the number of active physicians increased at an average annual rate of 3.3 percent per year between 1970 and 1986. In 1970 there were 150 active physicians per 100,000 persons as compared with 212 active physicians per 100,000 persons in 1986. That is, in 1970 there were approximately 669 persons per active physician as compared with 472 in 1986, a decrease of 29 percent.

The specialty composition of the physician population also changed during the period from 1970 to 1986. As illustrated in Table 3.1, the growth in some specialties significantly outpaced the overall growth in physician supply while the number of physicians in some other specialties actually declined over the 16-year period. Specialties that grew very rapidly include:

☐ Diagnostic Radiology (605%);

☐ Gastroenterology (222%);

*The population base for this calculation excludes inactive physicians and physicians with unknown addresses.

Table 3.1

Specialty	Percent	Specialty	Percent
Aerospace Medicine	−44.9	Occupational Medicine	−1.7
Allergy	−13.8	Ophthalmology	52.9
Anesthesiology	113.1	Orthopedic Surgery	83.6
Cardiovascular Disease	118.6	Otolaryngology	40.1
Child Psychiatry	85.6	Pathology	53.8
Colon and Rectal Surgery	25.2	Pediatrics	103.5
Dermatology	70.4	Pediatric Allergy	−4.6
Diagnostic Radiology	604.8	Pediatric Cardiology	78.2
Forensic Pathology	73.0	Physical Med./Rehab.	138.7
Gastroenterology	221.8	Plastic Surgery	161.6
General/Family Practice	16.8	Psychiatry	54.8
General Prev. Medicine	16.5	Public Health	−33.6
General Surgery	25.0	Pulmonary Diseases	136.0
Internal Medicine	118.1	Therapeutic Radiology	183.9
Neurology	168.8	Thoracic Surgery	16.9
Neurological Surgery	60.0	Urology	55.0
Obstetrics & Gynecology	66.2		

Percentage Change in Selected Physician Specialties 1970-1986

*Calculations exclude physicians who are not classified, inactive, or have an unknown address.

Source: Roback G, Randolph L, Seidman B, Mead D: *Physician Characteristics and Distribution in the U.S., 1987 Edition,* American Medical Association, 1987.

□ Therapeutic Radiology (184%); and

□ Neurology (169%).

Specialties with a declining number of practitioners over the period 1970-1986 include:

□ Aerospace Medicine (−45%);

□ Public Health (−34%); and

□ Allergy (−14%).

The changing specialty composition of the physician population is the result of a complex interaction among a number of factors. The changing employment opportunities for physicians in government have influenced the composition; the declining percentage of physicians in Aerospace Medicine and Public Health can be attributed to this factor. Advances in medical technology, such as those in Radiology, can alter the demand for physician services and induce changes in specialty composition. Changes in the demographic characteristics of physicians, particularly the growing number of female physicians, are related to specialty composition. For example, a higher proportion of female physicians choose Pediatrics as a specialty than do male physicians. Finally, the availability of residency positions also influences specialty composition.

In addition to the growing number of physicians, the number of specialties is also expanding. Since 1970, two new specialties in medicine were approved by the American Board of Medical Specialties: Nuclear Medicine and Emergency Medicine. Nuclear Medicine conferred its first certificates in 1972 and Emergency Medicine granted its first certificates in 1980. The number of physicians in Nuclear Medicine was 1,315 in 1986, while the number of physicians in Emergency Medicine was 12,297 in 1986. Recently, however, there has been little activity to approve new specialties.

There were only very slight changes in the professional activities of physicians during the period 1970 to 1986. As indicated by the figures in Table 3.2, the percent of physicians engaged in patient care activities increased slightly from 90 percent to 91 percent. The largest change in professional activity within the patient care category was the 3 percentage point increase in "office-based practice."*

---

*A physician in "office-based practice" is engaged primarily in patient care activities and is not employed by a hospital.

Table 3.2		
Major Professional Activity	1970	1986
Patient Care	89.5%	91.4%
Office Based Practice	61.8	64.7
Hospital Based Practice	27.7	26.7
Residents (all years)	16.5	17.5
Physician Staff	11.2	9.2
Medical Teaching	1.8	1.5
Administration	3.9	2.8
Research	3.8	3.5
Other	0.8	0.7

Percent Distribution of Physicians by Major Professional Activity, 1970 and 1986*

*The population base for the calculations excludes physicians who are inactive, not classified, or have unknown addresses.

Source: Roback G, Randolph L, Seidman B, Mead D: *Physician Characteristics and Distribution in the U.S., 1987 Edition*, American Medical Association, 1987.

The geographic distribution of physicians also changed between 1970 and 1986. In general, the changes in the geographic distribution of physicians have mirrored those of the general population. As illustrated in Table 3.3, the proportion of nonfederal, patient care physicians located in the Northeast and Midwest regions *decreased* between 1970 and 1986, while the proportion located in the South and West regions *increased*.

The diffusion of physicians into small cities and towns and into nonmetropolitan areas is another significant trend in the geographic distribution of physicians. By the end of the 1970s, nearly every town with a population of 2,500 or more had a physician or ready access to one. The number of nonfederal, patient-care physicians in nonmetropolitan areas increased by 46.5 percent between 1970 and 1986. Nevertheless, the overall proportion of nonfederal, patient-care physicians located in nonmetropolitan areas decreased from 14.6 percent to 12.3

Table 3.3

Distribution of
Nonfederal Patient
Care Physicians, by
Census Region,
1970 and 1986

Census Region	1970	1986
Northeast	30.9	26.3
Midwest	23.6	21.3
South	25.2	29.9
West	19.5	21.3
Possessions	0.9	1.2

Source: Roback G, Randolph L, Seidman B, Mead D: *Physician Characteristics and Distribution in the U.S., 1987 Edition,* American Medical Association, 1987.

percent between 1970 and 1986. This decline was almost entirely due to the decreasing proportion of general practitioners located in nonmetropolitan areas.

Finally, significant changes in other characteristics of the physician population between 1970 and 1986 include:

☐ The total number of female physicians increased from 25,40l to 86,670, a 241 percent increase; the percentage of female physicians in the total physician population increased from 7.6 percent to 15.2 percent;

☐ The total number of foreign medical graduates (FMGs) increased from 57,2l7 to 123,090, a 115 percent increase; the percentage of FMGs in the total physician population increased from 17.l percent to 21.6 percent; and

☐ The percentage of the physician population under age 45 increased from 51.7 percent to 53.6 percent.

Overall, 1970 through 1986 was a period of rapid increase in the supply of physician manpower and significant change in the characteristics of the physician population.

Economic Trends in
Medical Practice

Although individual physicians vary greatly in the nature of their practices, several key indicators—physicians' earnings, professional expenses, patient visits and fees—can be used to provide a general

Table 3.4

	Mean Net Income		Median Net Income		
	1977	1987	1977	1987	Mean and Median Net Income from Medical Practice, 1977 and 1987.
All Physicians	$60,400	$132,300	$55,000	$108,000	
Selected Specialties					
GP/FP	49,800	91,500	46,000	80,000	
IM	60,300	121,800	57,000	100,000	
Surgery	71,800	187,900	68,000	153,000	
Pediatrics	45,900	85,300	45,000	77,000	
Ob/Gyn	69,700	163,200	65,000	145,000	
Radiology	74,900	180,700	72,000	170,000	
Psychiatry	47,500	102,700	45,000	90,000	
Anesthesiology	65,900	163,100	62,000	150,000	

Definitions: Mean = arithmetic average; Median = midpoint of a distribution, i.e., half of the respondents are below that value and half are above that value.

Source: Gonzalez ML, Emmons DW (Editors): Socioeconomic Characteristics of Medical Practice 1988, American Medical Association, 1988.

perspective on the recent economic experiences of physicians.

Income

The average income of practicing physicians increased from $60,400 in 1977 to $132,300 in 1987. Adjusting for inflation, physicians real net incomes rose at an annual rate of 1.6 percent between 1977 and 1987. However, because the distribution of incomes is not symmetrical, mean or average net income may not indicate "what the average physician earns." For such purposes, median net income may be a better measure of the average physician's income.

As shown in Table 3.4, the median net income of practicing physicians increased from $55,000 in 1977 to $108,000 in 1987 for an average annual rate of growth of 7.0 percent. However, the median real (inflation adjusted) net income of physicians increased at an average

Table 3.5

Mean and Median Professional Expenses, 1977 and 1987

	Mean Expenses		Average Annual % Change	Median Expenses		Average Annual % Change
	1977	1987		1977	1987	
All Physicians*	$44,600	$123,700	10.7%	$35,000	$99,000	11.0%
Specialties						
GP/FP	44,700	121,200	10.5	39,000	96,000	9.4
IM	43,800	117,800	10.4	36,000	100,000	10.8
Surg.	58,200	164,700	11.0	45,000	133,000	11.4
Ped.	36,700	100,200	10.6	35,000	89,000	9.8
Ob/Gyn	61,500	173,200	10.9	50,000	149,000	11.5

*Includes other specialties not listed individually.

Source:Gonzalez ML, Emmons DW (Editors): *Socioeconomic Characteristics of Medical Practice 1987,* American Medical Association, 1987.

rate of only 0.5 percent per year between 1977 and 1987.

General and family practice physicians, internists, and pediatricians experienced decreases in real median net income. The average annual decline in real median incomes of general and family practitioners was 0.8 percent, compared with an average annual decline of 0.7 percent for internists and 0.9 percent for pediatricians. Conversely, the real median net incomes of radiologists, surgeons, and anesthesiologists *increased* at average yearly rates of 2.3, 1.8, and 2.6 percent, respectively.

Professional Expenses

The slow growth in physicians' real net incomes can be attributed, in part, to rapidly increasing professional expenses. As shown in Table 3.5, mean professional expenses rose from $44,600 in 1977 to $123,700 in 1987. Median total professional expenses increased from $35,000 in 1977 to $99,000 in 1987, an average annual rate of increase of 11 percent. This rate of growth exceeded both the rate of inflation and

Table 3.6

	Average Premiums (In thousands)			Percent Increase	
	1984	1985	1986	1984-85	1985-86
All Physicians*	$ 8.4	$10.5	$12.8	25.0%	21.9%
Specialty Group					
General/Family Practice	4.6	6.8	7.3	47.8	7.4
Medical Specialties	4.5	5.6	6.9	24.4	23.2
Surgical Specialties	14.8	18.3	23.2	23.6	26.8
Other Specialties	6.5	7.7	9.4	18.5	22.1

Average
Professional
Liability Premiums,
1984-1986

*Includes other specialties not listed individually.

Source: Gonzalez ML, Emmons DW: *Socioeconomic Characteristics of Medical Practice 1987*, Chicago: American Medical Association, 1987.

of growth in net income. As a result, the share of average practice revenues devoted to meeting expenses increased from 42 percent in 1977 to 48 percent in 1987.

A combination of factors are responsible for the increasing cost of practicing medicine. General inflation has contributed to rising unit costs of labor and other resources employed by physicians in their practices. Advances in technology have changed the nature of resources physicians use and the settings in which they provide different types of diagnoses and treatment. Increased medical liability risk has resulted in higher liability insurance premiums.

Professional liability continues to be a great concern to physicians. As indicated in Table 3.6, average professional liability premiums increased by 25 percent from 1984 to 1985, and by 22 percent from 1985 to 1986. In 1986, professional liability premiums averaged $12,800 for all physicians. Surgical specialists paid an average of $23,200 for liability insurance, while physicians in medical specialties paid an average of $6,900 in premium expenses.

Table 3.7

Average Patient
Visits Per Week,
1976 and 1986*

	1976	1986	Percent Change
Total Patient Visits**	134.7	117.7	−13.1%
Office Visits	95.8	75.7	−21.0
Visits on Hospital Rounds	35.0	25.8	−26.3

* Includes visits in emergency rooms, outpatient clinics and at all other locations.

**Based on all specialties except Psychiatry, Radiology, Anesthesiology and Pathology.

Source:Gonzalez ML, Emmons DW (Editors): *Socioeconomic Characteristics of Medical Practice 1987,* American Medical Association, 1987.

The rate of increase in professional liability premiums has varied by specialty. Premiums for physicians in General/Family Practice increased by 48 percent between 1984 and 1985, while premiums for surgical specialists rose by 24 percent. But between 1985 and 1986, premiums for General/Family practitioners increased by 7 percent, while premiums for surgical specialists rose by 27 percent.

Patient Visits

The decline in patient visits per physician, indicated in Table 3.7, is consistent with the generally expected effect of an increasing supply of physicians. Average total patient visits decreased by 13 percent from 135 per week in 1976 to 118 per week in 1986. Office visits decreased from an average of 96 per week in 1976 to 76 per week in 1986, a 21 percent decrease. Visits on hospital rounds decreased an average of 26 percent over this same period.

It should be noted that the information on visits excludes physicians in Psychiatry, Radiology, Anesthesiology and Pathology because visits are not a good measure of utilization for these specialties. Further, visits generally are an imperfect measure of utilization of physicians' services since patient visits vary in qualitative aspects and, perhaps, over time.

Physicians' Fees

Physicians' fees for various services have risen over the past decade.

Table 3.8

	1976	1986	Average Annual Percent Change
All Physicians*	$13.55	$30.10	8.3%
Specialties			
General/Family Practice	10.63	23.48	8.2
Internal Medicine	15.70	34.03	8.0
Surgery	13.93	29.66	7.9
Pediatrics	12.46	27.37	8.2
Obstetrics/Gynecology	15.39	34.81	8.5

Average Physician Fee for an Office Visit with an Established Patient, 1976 and 1986

*Includes all specialties except psychiatry, radiology, anesthesiology and pathology.

Source:Gonzalez ML, Emmons DW (Editors): Socioeconomic Characteristics of Medical Practice 1987, American Medical Association, 1987.

But when compared to the rate of change in the general price level, physicians' fees have not increased dramatically. For example, as shown in Table 3.8, the average fee for an office visit with an established patient, the most frequent single service provided by physicians, increased at an average annual rate of 8.3 percent from 1976 to 1986. While comparisons to changes in the Consumer Price Index are imperfect, it is interesting to note that the rate of increase in the average fee for an office visit with an established patient exceeded that of general inflation by only 1.5 percent.

In recent years there have been an increasing number of restrictions imposed by the federal government on the amount that physicians may charge and be reimbursed for services provided to Medicare beneficiaries.

□ In 1969, the prevailing charge was lowered from the 90th percentile to the 83rd percentile of customary charges.

□ In 1970, the prevailing charge was lowered to the 75th percentile of customary charges.

□ From August 1971 to May 1974, wage and price controls were imposed on physicians' fees.

□ In 1972, an economic index was imposed to limit the increase in prevailing charges.

□ In 1976, the economic index was used to set the prevailing charge limits, using fee screens from 1973, which were based on physicians' charges from 1971.

□ In 1984, legislation froze physicians' charges. The freeze was extended through March 1986.

□ In 1986, "non-participating" physicians (those who do not accept assignment for all Medicare patients) had their fees frozen throughout the year.

□ In 1987, the fee freeze of the previous year was replaced with a complex and graduated system of charge limitations for "non-participating" physicians known as MAACs (Maximum Allowable Actual Charge).

□ In 1987, a provision went into effect which stipulates that physicians who do not accept assignment on Medicare claims may be required to reimburse their patients for charges collected on services that Medicare determines to be "medically unnecessary."

□ In 1988, reductions in the prevailing charge levels for the following procedures were mandated: cataract surgery, coronary artery bypass surgery, total hip replacement, transurethral resection of the prostate, suprapubic prostatectomy, diagnostic and/or therapeutic dilation and curretage, bronchoscopy, knee arthroscopy, knee arthroplasty, pacemaker implantation, upper gastrointestinal endoscopy, and carpal tunnel repair.

The federal government is studying more extensive revisions in the reimbursement for services provided by physicians under Medicare. Proposals have been made to add Radiologists, Anesthesiologists, and Pathologists to hospital-based Medicare DRGs, as well as for develop-

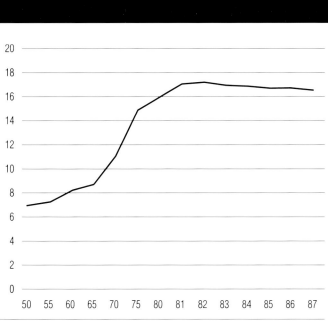

Figure 3.1

First Year
Medical Students
(in thousands)

Source: Medical Education in the United States, *JAMA*, various issues.

ing DRGs for other physicians. Congress is also considering the adoption of an indemnity reimbursement system based on a Relative Value Scale (RVS).

Among the major factors affecting the future supply of physicians and physicians' services are the current trends in undergraduate and graduate medical education. From these trends, and assuming certain rates of mortality and retirement, projections can be made of the future supply of physicians.

Projected Trends
in Physician
Manpower

Undergraduate Medical Education

Trends in medical education play a key role in the future supply of physicians. As indicated in Figure 3.1, the number of first-year medical students increased rapidly during the 1970s.

The apex of first-year enrollment occurred in 1981-82, when a total of 17,320 first-year students were seated. Since 1981-82, however, the first-year enrollment has been falling. In 1986-87, 16,779 students were enrolled in the first year of medical school.

One factor affecting medical school enrollment is the falling number of applicants. In 1981-82, approximately 36,700 individuals applied for medical school. By 1986-87, this number had fallen to 31,300, a decrease of about 15 percent.

One of the factors reducing the number of applicants to medical school may be the rising debt load of medical students. Average tuition in public medical schools has risen almost eightfold, from $478 in 1960 to $3959 in 1986. As a result of the rising cost of an undergraduate medical education, 82 percent of medical school graduates were in debt in 1986. The average debt was $33,500, but 17 percent had debts of more than $50,000. If other factors remain constant, and if debt loads continue to increase, the supply of medical school applicants may continue to fall.

Graduate Medical Education

A second factor affecting the future supply of physicians' services is the changing environment of graduate medical education. In 1987, there were 6,332 accredited residency training programs in the United States. Internal medicine had the largest number of programs, and approximately 27 percent of all residents were in programs for Internal Medicine. Surgery (general, pediatric, vascular) had almost 8,000 residents, and Pediatrics had 6,500 residents.

The sex composition of resident physicians is changing. Women residents are increasing in numbers and percentage. In 1977, 15 percent of residents were women; by 1987, 28 percent were women. According to the 1987 medical education report in JAMA, women residents are located in all specialties except Chemical Pathology and Medical Microbiology. About 40 percent of women residents are training in Internal Medicine or Pediatrics. Another 29 percent of women residents are in Obstetrics/Gynecology programs.

Foreign medical graduates are a declining influence in graduate residency programs. As indicated in Table 3.9, the number of FMGs in

	1985	1986	1987	**Table 3.9**
Sex				Number of
Male	54,952	56,069	58,787	Residents by Sex and Country of
Female	19,562	20,746	22,623	Graduation,
Country of Graduation				1985-1987
United States	62,005	64,780	68,698	
Foreign	12,509	12,035	12,712	

Source: Crowley AE, Etzel SI, Shaw HA: Graduate Medical Education in the United States, JAMA, August 28, 1987.

residency programs fell from 12,509 in 1985 to 12,712 in 1987.

These trends in the demographic characteristics of residents indicate that the future supply of physicians will be composed of more women and fewer foreign medical graduates.

Future Supply of Physicians

Combining the trends in undergraduate and graduate medical education with trends in the retirement and death of physicians, the AMA Center for Health Policy Research has projected future trends in physician manpower. In 1986, there were 519,411 active physicians in the United States. As indicated in Table 3.10, the Center projects that there will be approximately 633,200 active physicians in the year 2000.

The Center also projects that the specialty composition of the physician population will continue to change. As indicated in Table 3.10, the growth in some specialties is projected to significantly outpace the overall growth in physician supply, while the number of physicians in some other specialties is expected to increase slowly. Based on the current and projected demographic characteristics of the physician population, specialties that are projected to increase the fastest between 1986 and 2000 include:

☐ Emergency Medicine (55.2%);

Table 3.10

Projected Physician
Population by
Specialty, Sex
(Best Projection)

	1986	1990	2000	2010	1986-2000 % Change
Total Population	519,411	560,800	633,200	676,700	21.9%
General/Family Practice	68,437	70,900	74,600	77,800	9.0
General Internal Medicine	71,879	78,900	92,500	102,100	28.7
Medical Subspecialties	49,249	56,100	69,600	79,100	41.4
General Surgery	32,859	34,000	34,900	34,700	6.2
Surgical Subspecialties	66,643	71,200	77,200	78,800	15.8
Pediatrics	38,631	43,100	52,500	59,100	35.8
Obstetrics/Gynecology	31,882	34,400	39,100	42,100	22.7
Radiology	24,073	26,500	30,600	32,900	27.3
Psychiatry	37,440	39,400	42,100	42,800	12.4
Anesthesiology	23,705	26,000	32,200	35,700	35.4
Pathology	16,387	17,100	17,900	17,600	9.1
Emergency Medicine	12,343	14,600	19,200	22,500	55.2
Sex					
Male	439,805	460,600	480,400	477,800	9.2
Female	79,606	100,300	152,700	198,900	91.9

Source:WD Marder, PR Kletke, AB Silberger, RJ Wilke: *Physician Supply and Utilization by Specialty: Trends and Projections.* Chicago, American Medical Association, February 1988.

☐ Internal Medicine Subspecialties (53.8%); and

☐ Pediatrics (35.8%).

The specialties projected to grow at a slower than average pace include:

☐ General Surgery (6.2%);

☐ General/Family Practice (9.0%); and

☐ Pathology (9.1%).

Obstetrics/Gynecology is projected to grow at approximately the

Table 3.11

	1986	2000	1986-2000	Nonphysician
	(In thousands)		% Change	Health Care Workers
Total U.S. Employment	111,623	133,030	19%	
Dentists	151	196	30	
Dietitians	40	54	35	
Optometrists	37	55	49	
Pharmacists	151	187	24	
Physician Assistants	26	41	58	
Registered Nurses	1,406	2,018	44	
Occupational Therapists	29	45	55	
Physical Therapists	61	115	89	
Respiratory Therapists	56	76	36	
Medical Assistants	132	251	90	
Nursing Aides	1,312	1,750	33	
Health Technicians	1,598	2,261	41	

Source: A Look at Occupational Employment Trends to the Year 2000. *Monthly Labor Review*. September, 1987.

same pace as the overall physician supply.

Another significant change, as mentioned above, is the rapid growth in the number of women physicians. The number of women physicians is projected to increase from 79,606 in 1986 to 152,700 in 2000, an increase of 91.9 percent. The proportion of women physicians is expected to increase from approximately 15 percent of the physician supply in 1986 to almost 24 percent of the total supply in 2000.

The supply of health resources is also determined by the number of nonphysician health care personnel. Employment for health professionals is projected to grow rapidly. With the exception of the hospital sector, job growth in health care is expected to be among the fastest in the U.S. economy.

Trends in
Nonphysician
Health
Manpower

A number of health occupations, besides medicine, are projected to grow faster than the average for total employment in the United States. Total U.S. employment is projected to increase by 19 percent between 1986 and 2000. Table 3.11 indicates that health care employment will rise from a low 24 percent for pharmacists to a high of around 90 percent for physical therapists and medical assistants between 1986 and 2000.

The projections of employment in Table 3.11, however, do not indicate the current environment of health care employment. In particular, there is currently a perceived shortage of nurses and certain other allied health personnel in the United States. The shortage of bedside nurses is considered a factor in the closure of critical care units and medical/surgical units in many areas of the United States. In a recent survey, nursing vacancies were reported in most hospitals, and only 17.6% of hospitals surveyed reported having no RN vacancies in 1986-1987.

Physicians, nurses and allied health personnel comprise part of the supply of health care resources available in the United States. However, other factors affect the supply of health care resources, including:

☐ The numbers and types of health care delivery systems;

☐ Methods of financing health care resources.

Hospitals

The supply of hospital resources has been changing in recent years. The number of community hospitals has been decreasing, but the number of community hospital beds is increasing. Over the 1976-86 period:

☐ The number of community hospitals decreased by 3.1 percent;

☐ The supply of community hospital beds increased by 2.3 percent; and

☐ The number of community hospital personnel increased by 22.2 percent.

The number of admissions to community hospitals fell by 4.7 percent, and the number of inpatient days fell by 12.0 percent. Table 3.12

presents data on trends in the characteristics of the three principal types of community hospitals (nongovernmental, investor owned, and state and local governmental) over the 1976-86 period.

In addition to increasing in bed size, community hospitals have expanded the scope and intensity of services provided. Community hospital services are increasingly provided in an outpatient setting. Outpatient visits at community hospitals increased by 15.2 percent between 1976 and 1986, as compared to a 12.0 percent decrease in inpatient days.

There has been a trend towards more services offered in community hospitals, as indicated by the expansion of facilities and services available at community hospitals. In 1986, for example, 93.3 percent of community hospitals offered ambulatory surgical services, 86.2 percent offered ultrasound services, 72.0 provided health promotion services, and 60.3 percent had a CT scanner.

Investor-owned (for-profit) community hospitals have become much more similar to other community hospitals in recent years. Nevertheless, relative to other community hospitals, for-profit hospitals generally are smaller, employ fewer personnel per patient, have a shorter average length of stay for inpatient cases, and have a lower occupancy rate. Although the number of investor-owned hospitals has been increasing only slightly, the influence of investor-owned companies has been growing through management contracts. According to the Federation of American Health Systems, the number of U.S. not-for-profit hospitals managed under contract by investor-owned companies increased from 127 to 325 between 1976 and 1984, a 155.9 percent increase in eight years.The geographic distribution of community hospital resources has also been changing. As suggested by the figures presented in Table 3.13, the geographic distribution of hospital resources has been following the pattern of population movement with the exception of hospitals in the West, which may reflect the consolidation of smaller

Table 3.12

Selected Measures
in Community
Hospitals,
1976 and 1985-86

Measure	Year			% Change	
	1976	1985	1986	1976-86	1985-86
Hospitals	5,857	5,732	5,678	−3.1%	−0.9%
Beds (000s)	956	1,001	978	2.3	−2.2
Average number of beds per hospital	163	175	172	5.5	−1.3
Admissions (000s)	33,979	33,449	32,379	−4.7	−3.2
Average daily census (000s)	713	649	629	−11.8	−3.1
Average length of stay, days	7.7	7.1	7.1	−7.7	0.2
Inpatient days (000s)	260,742	236,619	229,448	−12.0	−3.0
Occupancy, percent	74.6	64.8	64.3	−13.8	−0.9
Surgical operations (000s)	16,832	20,113	20,469	21.6	1.8
Bassinets (000s)[a]	82	75	74	−10.5	−1.6
Births (000s)[a]	2,962	3,521	3,584	21.0	1.8
Outpatient visits (000s)[b]	201,247	218,716	231,912	15.2	6.0

Source: American Hospital Association, *Hospital Statistics, 1987 Edition,* 1987.

a Based only on hospitals reporting newborn data.

b Based only on hospitals reporting outpatient data.

investor-owned hospitals in that region.

Trends in Other Delivery Systems

The growth of other health care delivery systems in recent years is one reflection of a rapidly changing health care environment. Increasing competition, combined with the cost containment environment, has led to the proliferation of group medical practices, health maintenance organizations, preferred provider organizations, ambulatory surgery centers, and emergency centers. The proliferation of these delivery systems could significantly affect the cost of, access to, and quality of medical care.

As table 3.14 indicates, the number of group practices has increased from 10,762 in 1980 to 17,516 in 1987, an annual increase of 7.2

Table 3.13

Census Division	1976	1986	Percent Change	Population Change 1975-1985
Total Community Hospitals	5,857	5,678	−3.1%	
Census Division				
Northeast	922	836	−9.3	0.9
Midwest	1,722	1,647	−4.4	2.3
South	2,105	2,134	1.4	17.7
West	1,108	1,061	−4.2	23.9

Distribution of Community Hospitals, by region, 1976 and 1986

Sources: American Hospital Association, *Hospital Statistics 1987.* Bureau of the Census, *Statistical Abstract of the United States, 1987,* Table 25.

Table 3.14

Groups	1980	1984	1987
Groups	10,762	15,485	17,516
Groups 100+	76	158	168
Physician Positions in all Groups	88,290	140,392	155,051
Physician Positions in Groups 100+	18,899	41,342	45,336
Ratio Positions in Large Groups to Positions in Groups	21.4	29.4	29.2

Group Practices in the US

Source: AMA Department of Survey and Data Resources.

percent. Large group practices with over 100 physicians have increased from 76 in 1980 to 168 in 1987, an annual increase of 12.0 percent. The percentage of group practice positions in large group practices increased from 21 percent in 1980 to 29 percent in 1984. Since that time, the percentage of group practice positions in large group practices has remained at the 29 percent level.

Health maintenance organizations (HMOs) have been growing rapidly. HMOs provide health care services to an enrolled population for a predetermined and fixed periodic payment. As indicated in table 3.15,

Table 3.15

Growth in HMOs,
1982-1987

Year	Number	Percent Change	Enrollment in Millions	Percent Change
1982	265		10.8	
1983	280	5.7	12.5	15.7
1984	306	9.3	15.1	20.8
1985	393	28.4	18.9	25.2
1986	595	51.4	23.7	25.4
1987	662	11.3	28.6	20.7

Source: InterStudy: *The Interstudy Edge*, Fall 1987.

the number of HMOs has grown rapidly through 1986. In 1987, however, the growth in HMOs slowed considerably. Despite the recent slowdown in the number of HMOs, enrollment in HMOs has increased by over 20 percent per year since 1983. In 1987, approximately 8.5 percent of the US population were enrolled in HMOs. A survey by the AMA Center for Health Policy Research estimates that more than 42 percent of physicians in 1986 had a contract with an HMO.

There are several forms of HMOs.

☐ Staff Model delivers health care services through a physician group controlled by the HMO unit.

☐ Group Model delivers health care services through an independent physician group.

☐ Network Model delivers health care services through several physician groups.

☐ Independent Practice Association (IPA) Model delivers health care services through independently practicing physicians.

Group model HMOs dominated the HMO market during the early 1980s. However, this trend is beginning to change. As indicated in table 3.16, 44 percent of the HMO enrollment received care in group model HMOs in 1984. However, the dominant HMO form has become the

Table 3.16

Total Enrollment (In millions)	1984	1985	1986	1987	1988
	15.3	18.9	23.6	28.6	31.0
Proportion in:					
Staff Model	14%	14%	13%	11%	12%
Group Model	44	34	30	25	26
Network Model	23	27	21	24	20
Independent Practice Association (IPA)	19	25	36	40	42

Enrollment in Health Maintenance Organizations (HMOs) by Model Type, 1984-1988

Note: All statistics for June of indicated years, except for 1988 when March is reported.

Source: Interstudy

Independent Practice Association, with 42 percent of the total HMO enrollment in 1988. Staff model HMOs and Network model HMOs, combined, have represented about one-third of the HMO enrollment between 1984 and 1988.

In addition to IPAs, open-ended HMOs are beginning to increase in numbers. These HMOs are a hybrid form of health insurance, combining features of HMO insurance with indemnity coverage. Under these plans, a patient has some flexibility to choose whether to use the HMO services or the indemnity service. Receiving care under the indemnity provisions of the plan typically involves increased patient cost-sharing however. In 1987, InterStudy, a consulting firm for HMOs, determined that there were 22 HMOs reporting open-ended enrollment, which covered over 330,000 individuals.

Preferred Provider Organizations (PPOs) continue to represent a significant alternative delivery model. PPOs are associations of physicians and hospitals that contract with employers and insurers to provide health care services on a negotiated fee-for-service basis. The PPO arrangement allows subscribers to choose any provider for care. If the subscriber, however, chooses a provider outside the PPO plan, that subscriber is usually required to pay a higher deductible and copayment.

Table 3.17

The Number of
Operational PPOs

Year	Number	Percent Change From Previous Year
1981	27	
1982	45	66.7%
1983	107	137.8
1984	223	108.4
1985	379	70.0
1986	493	30.1
1987	535	8.5

Source: American Medical Care and Review Association: *Directory of Preferred Provider Organizations and the Industry Report on PPO Development,* Bethesda, American Medical Care and Review Association, June 1987.

The growth in the number of PPOs was rapid throughout the early and mid-1980s, but recently has shown signs of slowing. As indicated in Table 3.17, there were 45 operational PPOs in 1982. The number of PPOs increased to 223 in 1984 and to 493 in 1986. In 1987, there were 535 operational PPOs in the United States.

The AMA Center for Health Policy Research estimates that about 38 percent of physicians had some type of a contractual arrangement with a PPO in 1986. The number of PPO contracts with physicians exceeded 654,000 in 1987. Thus, many physicians have signed contracts with more than one PPO. Early surveys by the AMA Center found that many physicians contracted with PPOs but did not receive revenues from them. However, between 1984 and 1986, the proportion of physicians with PPO contracts who reported that they received no revenues from their contracts fell from 26.1 percent to 12.4 percent.

As indicated in Table 3.18, physicians, either alone or in joint venture, are sponsors of 218 operational or preoperational PPOs. Hospitals and physicians have sponsored almost half of the currently existing PPOs,

	Number	Percent of Total	**Table 3.18**
			PPO Sponsorship
Hospitals and Physicians	282	49.5	Operational (535)
Hospitals	64	11.2	Preoperational (35)
Hospital-Physician Joint Ventures	113	19.8	
Physicians	105	18.4	
Insurance Companies	180	31.6	
Blue Cross/Blue Shield Plans	59	10.4	
Other Insurance Co.	121	21.1	
Investors	47	8.2	
Third Party Administrators	25	4.4	
HMOs	18	3.2	
Others	18	3.2	

Source: American Medical Care and Review Association: *Directory of Preferred Provider Organizations and the Industry Report on PPO Development,* Bethesda, American Medical Care and Review Association, June 1987.

insurance companies have sponsored less than one-third of the PPOs, and investors comprise only 8 percent of the sponsors.

The geographic distribution of PPOs is uneven. Almost 19 percent of PPOs are located in the state of California. As a result, over one-third of all PPOs are located in the West region. As indicated in Table 3.19, the South has 23 percent of the PPOs, the Northeast has 22 percent, and the Midwest has 20 percent.

Other delivery systems increasing in numbers are freestanding ambulatory care centers and emergency centers. Although almost all hospitals provide ambulatory surgery, the Freestanding Ambulatory Surgical Association estimates that there will be approximately 830 independent ambulatory surgery centers by 1990. And, the number of freestanding emergency centers is expected to increase from 3,000 in 1985 to 5,000 by 1990.

Table 3.19

	PPOs	Percent of Total
Northeast	128	22.4
South	151	26.5
Midwest	117	20.5
West	194	34.0
Total	570	100.0

Regional Distribution of Operational and Preoperational PPOs

Source: American Medical Care and Review Association: *Directory of Preferred Provider Organizations and the Industry Report on PPO Development,* Bethesda, American Medical Care and Review Association, June 1987.

4

Changing
Roles in the
Health Sector

This chapter discusses the roles of the key participants in the health sector—government, business, labor, insurers, consumers, hospitals, and organized medicine. Their historical roles and recent changes in those roles are identified and analyzed.

Key Participants

Government

The financial influence of the federal government on health care has become substantial. Table 4.1 indicates that federal health expenditures as a percentage of total health care expenditures has increased dramatically. As a result, the federal government has considerable influence in the health care environment of today. Currently, about 30 cents of every health dollar is spent by the federal government.

Table 4.1

Health Expenditures
in the United States

Year	National Health Expenditures*	Federal Health Expenditures*	Federal Share of Total Health Expenditures
1965	$41.9	$5.5	13.1%
1970	75.0	17.7	23.6
1975	132.7	37.0	28.0
1980	248.1	71.0	28.6
1985	422.6	124.5	29.5
1990	647.3	195.5	30.2
1995	999.1	317.7	31.8
2000	1,529.3	498.6	32.6

Source: National Health Expenditures, 1986-2000. *Health Care Financing Review,* Summer 1987. *Amounts in billions.

Prior to the end of World War II, the federal government did not exert much leadership in the health care system. As the war stimulated growth in medical technology and increased the demand for health care services, a wide-spread perception developed that the nation's hospitals needed to be modernized and expanded. In response to this perception, the government embarked on a course of direct intervention in the health care system with the passage of the Hill-Burton Act. This program provided loans and grants to the states, which funneled them to hospitals for the construction of facilities, and thereby provided for the wide-scale implementation of the new medical knowledge gained during the war. As part of the program, institutions involved had to establish minimum operational standards and states were asked to develop planning methodologies. In essence, government became a partner in providing medical care resources to the public.

During the decades of the 1960s and 1970s, government involvement in health care continued to expand. The federal government initiated programs to correct a perceived shortage of health professionals and to provide reimbursement for care provided to elderly and indigent individuals.

To provide reimbursement for care provided to the elderly and indigent, Congress enacted the Medicare and Medicaid laws, making government a major financer of medical care. However, government concern over providing the appropriate amount of care required tying participation in Medicare reimbursement to utilization review criteria. As a result, the behavior of providers became increasingly subject to the scrutiny of various public health agencies.

As many of the well-intentioned government health care programs matured, public officials became acutely aware that their projections about utilization, supply, and costs of health services were inaccurate. As organized medicine had predicted, the governmental payouts for these programs were consuming a larger percentage of public budgets than anticipated. The public sector reacted by looking for ways to curb its total spending for health programs.

As the 1980s began, economists and policymakers debated the wisdom of the regulatory approach to cost containment. Many believed that regulation was not meeting its goals. Some argued for a decreased reliance on direct regulation and increased reliance upon market forces to determine the proper level of health care expenditures. This "pro competition" group introduced a number of pieces of legislation intended to induce patients to economize in making their health care consumption decisions.

The federal government has promoted development of a more competitive health care market by shifting more responsibility for medical care to state and local governments, de-emphasizing centralized health planning, and taking a less active role in supply activities. Further, the federal government introduced prospective pricing for hospital services under Medicare as a means of shifting responsibility for cost restraint to hospital service providers.

As the largest purchaser of health care, government has attempted to become a more "prudent buyer" by exerting more control over the amount paid for services. Historically, the retrospective cost method of reimbursing hospitals and the customary and prevailing charge method of paying for professional services placed the federal government in the role of "price-taker." Recent federal legislation, aimed at controlling Medicare costs, has been enacted in an attempt to reposition the government in the role of "price-maker."

Another strategy of the federal government to reduce its health care outlays is to shift responsibility for health care to state and local governments. In turn, state governments have begun exploring options to increase the extent of health expense protection. One option receiving particular attention involves some form of mandate for employers to provide health insurance coverage for their employees. A recent Massachusetts law, which takes this approach, is being watched carefully by other states and may become a model for some states.

In summary, the role of government in the health sector has undergone a number of evolutionary steps since the end of World War II.

Beginning as a passive observer, the federal government first intervened to encourage the development of more hospital resources. Next, programs were developed to increase the supply of health care services and improve access to health care. As costs and utilization increased, government turned to directly regulating the delivery of health care. When direct regulation did not work, the government began to intervene to encourage more economic competition and to restrict payment under government programs. Several comments can be made about this progression:

☐ The financial outlay of government for health care has increased consistently.

☐ The scope and intensity of governmental attempts to modify the economic performance of the sector have increased as the costs of government health programs have increased.

☐ Every governmental attempt to modify the economic performance of the health sector has created new, unanticipated problems to which government has responded with new programs.

Although its direction may change again, governmental attempts to modify the economic performance of the health care sector are likely to continue. All levels of government cannot withdraw from their commitment to the provision of health care services to the poor, disadvantaged, and elderly individuals because governmental "promises" and programs in the health area have generated political expectations. However, budgetary problems at all levels of government make it increasingly difficult for these commitments to be fulfilled. The current strategy of the federal government is to alter the economic performance of the health care sector in order to contain health care expenditures. But, it can be argued that the federal government tends to focus on "symptoms" rather than fundamental problems in the health sector and, as a result, federal intervention almost always creates a new series of problems, which "require" new strategies of intervention.

Business

Until the 1940s, American industry played a passive role in the health care system. With the growth of labor unions and the acceptance of collective bargaining, health insurance began to be offered as an employee benefit. Business historically did not try to intervene in how these dollars were being spent because the expense was tax deductible as part of the cost of employing workers and the total payout was not a substantial part of business expense.

In recent years the attitude of corporate America has changed. A number of American industries now face declining demand for their products. Competition has become global and foreign competitors have the advantage of lower labor costs and increased governmental aid. American firms can no longer simply pass operating costs along to consumers via increased prices. American business leaders have become more cost conscious in order to preserve and enhance profits. They see that dollars saved as a result of reduced health premium expenses can have a substantial impact on business profits. As a result, business has adopted a more activist role in containing health care costs. Business activities in this area include:

Health Care Coalitions. There are approximately 113 organizations believed to be health care coalitions in the country, which include as members representatives of such interest groups as business, labor, physicians, hospitals, insurers, and government. They share information on costs and utilization and involve themselves in a wide variety of current issues, including substance abuse and quality of care.

Alternative Delivery Systems. Many businesses have embraced health maintenance organizations, individual practice associations, and preferred provider organizations. Some firms claim that they have experienced a reduction in premiums when significant numbers of employees enroll in these plans. A 1986 survey by the Business Roundtable, an association of business executives, found that 92

Figure 4.1

Alternative Delivery
Systems

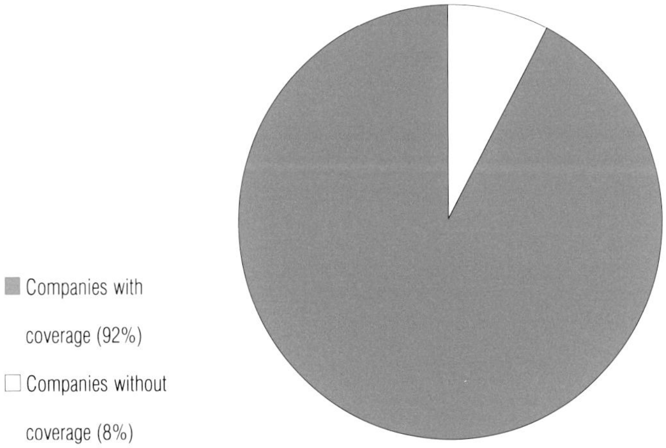

■ Companies with
  coverage (92%)

□ Companies without
  coverage (8%)

Source: Business Roundtable, 1987.

Table 4.1

	Percentage of Companies
Will Pay for Second Opinions	95%
Offer Financial Incentives for Second Opinions	80%
Do Not Provide for Second Opinions	5%

Reimbursement for
Second Surgical
Opinion

Source: Business Roundtable, 1987.

percent of the companies represented in the Roundtable offer coverage
for alternative delivery systems (see Figure 4.1).

Employee Education. Firms are attempting to develop programs to
educate employees on how to become "prudent buyers" and on
maintaining wellness (see Figure 4.2).

Second-Opinion Programs. Some firms are requiring that employees
seek a second surgical opinion for elective surgery (see Table 4.1).

Wellness Programs. Many firms have developed programs to
promote physical fitness, stop smoking, reduce body weight, and screen
for hypertension. While many of these programs have been implemented
without the benefit of cost/benefit analyses, many firms believe that

Figure 4.2

Employee Health
Education Programs

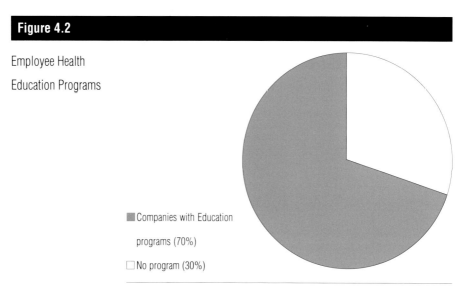

■ Companies with Education

   programs (70%)

□ No program (30%)

Source: Business Roundtable, 1987.

efforts to reduce the risk of disabling illnesses to their employees is a
worthwhile social and business investment.

Cost-Sharing. Cost-sharing requires employees to pay more of their
health costs out-of-pocket through the use of coinsurance and deductibles. Studies have shown that raising deductibles decreases utilization.
Some businesses offer a cash rebate for not using health insurance, and
others offer a variety of flexible benefit plans.

Self-Insurance Programs. More and more firms are self-insuring.
Financial reasons are the major factor cited by those companies that
self-insure. Self-insured plans are exempt from state health insurance
laws by virtue of the federal ERISA law.

Mandated Benefits. Two states, Hawaii and Massachusetts, have
mandated that employers contribute to the cost of health insurance for
their employees.

Labor

Labor leaders traditionally sought to increase tax-free benefits for
workers and improve accessibility to care, but did not attempt to
intervene in the health sector. As the pressure to contain health care
costs has mounted, coupled with declining union membership, labor's

Figure 4.3

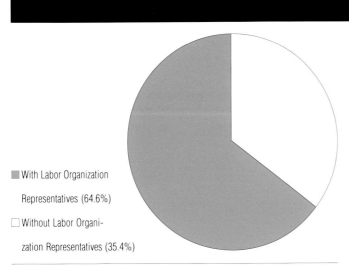

Coalitions with
Labor Organization
Representatives

■ With Labor Organization
   Representatives (64.6%)
☐ Without Labor Organi-
   zation Representatives (35.4%)

Source: American Hospital Association

role has shifted to include efforts to modify the economic performance
of the health sector. Organized labor remains committed to preserving
the health benefits it currently has, but has become active in promoting
cost containment efforts and educational programs that assist employees in making informed decisions. Labor has also become an active
participant in some health care coalitions, promoting many of industry's
goals to reduce health costs.

   Although labor's political and economic strength may appear to have
waned recently, it is a voice to be heard, particularly because of its
shared concern with business and other interest groups over the cost,
access, and quality of care issues in health care.

Insurers

Traditionally, third parties acted as "pass through" mechanisms for
health expenditures. They adopted a passive role with regard to the
economic performance of the health sector and with regard to physicians' practice patterns. The financial difficulties experienced by the
health insurance industry over the past decade have induced them to
adopt a more activist role in the health sector.

   The health insurance industry has recently experienced a poor financial performance. New and expensive medical technology, inflation in the health sector, and unexpected increases in utilization forced third parties to pay more for medical care than they anticipated when premiums were determined. Many commercial carriers are exploring new methods to more accurately anticipate utilization and to control their payouts. Some of these are:

□ Sponsoring HMOs.

□ Using selective contracting with certain providers.

□ Expanding coverage to include care in less expensive settings.

□ Incorporating more cost-sharing features in policies.

□ Identifying "outmoded" and experimental procedures for which third parties will not reimburse providers.

The driving forces behind the structural changes in the health insurance sector are rising health care prices and increased utilization. The level of health insurance premiums charged by Blue Cross/Blue Shield (BC/BS) and commercial insurance plans has risen rapidly in recent years. The upward trend in premiums has provided an incentive for individuals and businesses to search for ways to reduce their expenditures on health insurance coverage. The results have been an increase in the level of competition in the insurance sector and rapid growth in self-funded plans. Many employers have recently redesigned their benefit packages in an attempt to reduce business health insurance expenses.

There is, in a sense, a classic confrontation taking place between insurers and providers. Insurers believe they must use their provider contracts and reimbursement formulae to maintain control over costs and utilization, and to demonstrate to business and the public that they can provide adequate benefits at reasonable cost. Many providers, on the other hand, are attempting to free themselves from the constraints and rules imposed by insurance companies. Many physicians believe that third parties are beginning to interfere with medical decisions through the implementation and operation of preadmission review programs, second surgical opinion procedures, and other programs designed to restrain costs.

Patients

There seems to be no doubt that the general public is becoming increasingly aware of personal health issues. Public opinion polls show that Americans are more concerned with what they eat and drink and are more aware of the relationships between a variety of factors (i.e., smoking, exercise, stress) and their overall health status. Advances in communication technology have made detailed health information readily available to many Americans. Consequently, the general public is also becoming more familiar with and interested in health policy issues. It is likely that medical care consumers will play a more active role in making their own health care consumption decisions as well as the direction of society's health policy. Physicians can expect that patients will become less passive, and more questioning, about health care decisions. As consumers become better acquainted with health care concepts and more comfortable with participating in health care decision making, they may also become more likely to "shop" for their health care services more carefully, thus further increasing competitive forces in the medical care sector.

Hospitals

Recent developments within the health care delivery system have shaken the nation's hospitals. Some of these developments are:

☐ Utilization of inpatient services is either declining or remaining constant on a nationwide basis. Excess capacity exists in many institutions.

☐ Tighter reimbursement schemes including rate review, prospective pricing, and contracted discounts are adversely affecting the surpluses (or profits) of hospitals. A smaller surplus limits an institution's ability to acquire capital funding for modernization and expansion.

□ Alternative delivery systems have begun to compete with a variety of hospital services. These include birthing centers, emergicenters, and surgicenters. Some hospitals are finding it difficult to compete on a price basis with the new delivery systems.

□ The hospital sector is undergoing consolidation—the number of community hospitals is changing only slightly, while community hospital size is increasing.

□ Managerial control of hospitals is changing—the number of hospitals in multi-hospital systems is increasing and the influence of for-profit hospitals is increasing.

□ Rural hospitals are forming regional alliances to remain viable.

Economic pressures are the driving force behind the changing structure of the hospital sector. Hospital costs and charges have been growing rapidly for decades. As pressures to contain charges have increased and the government has imposed more and more constraints on Medicare and Medicaid reimbursement of hospitals, the hospital sector has undergone structural change in order to increase efficiency and to diversify the sources of hospital revenues. The system of reimbursing hospitals by diagnosis-related groups (DRGs) for Medicare patients is creating economic pressures that will further encourage more hospitals to restructure and to expand their services.

Hospitals are reacting to these changes by changing their roles. They are becoming active competitors for the health care dollar. In some cases, they are becoming direct competitors with physicians. Although physicians and hospitals are still dependent upon each other, economic pressures have forced hospitals to adopt more aggressive and competitive postures with regard to physicians.

Organized Medicine

Until the 1930s, organized medicine concentrated its efforts on the accreditation of educational institutions, the promotion of public health, the publication of scientific journals, the health education of the public, and the promotion of quality medical care. In the 1930s, medicine began to take a broader role in the medical care delivery system.

Changes in the national scene since the end of World War II, particularly the increasing involvement of government in health care, have caused an evolution in the role of organized medicine. Organized medicine has increasingly focused on representation of the medical profession on socioeconomic issues. The continuing attempts of government to alter the economic performance of the health sector suggest that this aspect of the role of organized medicine will continue to be important in the future.

Over time, organized medicine has been involved in a number of topical issues affecting physicians and their patients. Much energy has been devoted to the appraisal of new clinical techniques, the evaluation of drugs and devices, the investigation of claims and warnings, and the exposure of fraud. The successful campaign against alcohol advertising, the significant efforts to reduce the hazards of sports participation, and the current campaigns for a smoke-free society, are but a few of many examples of organized medicine's influence on public health.

As the parameters of medical technology, medical knowledge and medical capability have expanded, many ethical questions have been raised. Organized medicine has taken a leading role in addressing issues such as withdrawing life prolonging medical treatment, genetic engineering, and organ donation and transplantation. By providing a forum for physicians and other interested parties to come together and explore these and related ethical issues, organized medicine serves the interests of both the physician and his or her patients.

In addition to these ethical issues, related social policy issues have commanded the attention of organized medicine. The crisis in adolescent health, rising infant mortality rates, increased substance abuse, and the myriad of issues surrounding the AIDS epidemic are receiving careful consideration. The issues confronting society and the practice of medicine will become more complex and more demanding. The rising cost of health care and the subsequent efforts at cost containment will continue the debate over the allocation of health resources, ensuring access to needed medical care, and ensuring the provision of quality care. Organized medicine will continue to play a vital role in shaping a response to these challenges and determining health policy in the United States.

Some of the major issues that are expected to develop considerable discussion among these key participants in the health care sector during the coming years include the following.

Cost of Medical Care

The cost of medical care in the United States has been rising rapidly. The increase in the cost of medical care is due to a number of factors including a growing population, increasing prices for medical care goods and services, increasing intensity of services provided, and increasing prices in the general economy. The result of these myriad forces is that the health care sector is growing at a faster rate than the overall economy.

The increasing cost of health care has led to calls to contain health care costs. Many forces for change in the economy are either caused by rising health care costs or cause health care costs to rise.

Physician Reimbursement

In the 1970s and early 1980s, many cost containment programs were directed toward hospital costs. It is expected that the focus of these programs will shift toward containing physician costs in the future. The current system of reimbursing physicians under Medicare is considered inflationary. Thus, Congress has been looking at alternative reimbursement mechanisms, including most notably a capitation system and a fee schedule system.

Private third-party payors are keenly interested in any changes in physician reimbursement under Medicare and it is likely that some will institute similar reimbursement provisions.

Quality of Care Evaluation and Assurance

As government, business and other payors search for methods to reduce their health care costs, and as competition intensifies in the health care sector, efforts to preserve the quality of health care will become increasingly important. Pressures will grow for changes in delivery and financing systems which may present threats to quality of care. Public debate will increasingly focus on how to define and measure quality.

Quality is difficult to measure and even where measurements exist, they are often challenged as to their precision and application. Despite the difficulty in measuring quality of medical care, it is likely that quality measurement systems will increase substantially.

Professional Liability

Professional liability has been and continues to be an issue of considerable importance to the medical profession. Over one-third of all physicians in 1986 had been sued at least once in their career. However, professional liability concerns vary considerably by location. For years, the medical profession has been pushing for tort reform. Support for tort reform was also voiced by the nation's judiciary, in a survey of state and federal court judges. However, major challenges remain in reforming the tort system.

Shortage of Nurses

The shortage of nurses has become critical in many areas. Only 17.6 percent of hospitals surveyed reported having no RN vacancies in 1986-1987. The nursing shortage is disrupting bedside care and is impacting on the safety and effectiveness of medical services in hospitals. Innovative solutions to the problem of a shortage of bedside nurses will need to be implemented in order to preserve the quality of inpatient care.

Health Expense Protection for the Uninsured

An estimated 37 million individuals under age 65 are uninsured for health care costs. A number of proposals have been advanced to address this problem, including expansion of the Medicaid program, establishment of state risk pools, and providing incentives or mandates for businesses to provide insurance for their employees. In 1988, the Massachusetts legislature passed a mandated health care program to provide insurance to working people and their families. The Massachusetts plan also requires employers to contribute to a state pool that would provide insurance to the unemployed and to workers not protected by employer-provided health care insurance.

Legislators across the nation have begun to track the Massachusetts plan and some are drafting their own version of the mandated health care plan. Over a dozen states are expected to deal with this topic during 1989.

Long-Term Care

Issues in financing health care for elderly citizens continue to be at the forefront of national policy debate. Medicare has been expanded to include coverage for catastrophic health care costs. However, financing of long-term care services remains problematic.

One of the key impediments in discussions of long-term care policy are differences in defining precisely what constitutes long-term care. By its very nature, long-term care incorporates health care services and varying degrees of social services. Most analysts define long-term care to include physician care, physical, occupational and speech therapy, and occasional assistance in personal hygiene and activities of daily living as an extension of nursing care when necessitated by a chronic medical problem.

Estimates developed by the Washington-based consulting firm, ICF indicate that, during 1987, an estimated $36.3 billion was spent on long-term care services in the United States, of which nearly $18.8 billion was provided by public sources.

Despite the total amount of public dollars expended, long-term care costs continue to pose a major threat to the financial well-being of older persons. According to ICF projections, about 600,000 elderly persons admitted to nursing homes in 1988 had out-of-pocket expenditures of $5,000 or more and approximately 20 percent of these individuals had out-of-pocket expenses of over $50,000.

Some policy analysts believe that long-term care costs are a public responsibility and should be funded through a national program. Others contend that long-term care financing is a public-private responsibility. The financing of the costs of long-term care is likely to generate considerable debate in the coming years.

Acquired Immunodeficiency Syndrome (AIDS)

The AIDS epidemic can significantly alter the socioeconomic fabric of the United States. As of December 12, 1988, a total of 80,538 AIDS cases had been reported to the Centers for Disease Control; of these, 45,164 patients had died. It has been estimated that 1 to 1.5 million persons in the United States were infected with the AIDS virus as of June 1986.

AIDS is likely to be a leading cause of death in the United States by the early 1990s, adding about $4-6 billion in health care costs. While most groups agree with the need for AIDS research, differences arise over the financing of AIDS research. Further complicating the search for a potential AIDS vaccine is the shortage of animals for experimentation and the conscious efforts being made to impede the use of animals in biomedical research by vocal, well-financed activists.

5

Conclusions and
Implications

In the past decade, there has been rapid growth in physician manpower, significant advances in medical technologies, increased pressures on the hospital-physician relationship, the emergence of alternative delivery systems, and more aggressive health care cost containment activities.

There are several general themes or conclusions that can be drawn from the latest trends affecting medicine, including:

Theme 1. Cost pressures will continue to be the principal driving force underlying change in the medical care environment.

Many of the current trends in the environment can be traced, either directly or indirectly, to the cost issue. It is likely that rapid environmental change will persist until the cost issue is resolved in some manner. The key question is what type of change in the health care system will preserve the most crucial features of the current delivery system and also contain costs?

The growing proportion of the GNP allocated to health care means that the economic efficiency of the medical care sector will continue to be scrutinized and proposals to alter the economic performance of the sector will continue to emerge.

It is likely that the federal deficit will place added emphasis on the development of methods to contain federal health care costs.

If inflation and interest rates move upward, young physicians may be particularly affected. Large educational debt loads may place serious economic constraints on their practice choices. For example, economic considerations may encourage young physicians to accept salaried positions.

The shifting geographic pattern of medical resources will create upward pressure on medical care costs. As would be expected in a market economy, medical resources are moving in the same direction as the general population. Although this movement is desirable in order to provide the public with ready access to medical services, this trend does place upward pressure on costs, particularly hospital costs. Hospitals in areas with a declining population may have to run at an uneconomically low level of activity or may have to close entirely. In areas with a rapidly growing population, expensive new hospital facilities must be built. The net result may be an increase in the costs of providing the public with access to hospital facilities.

The professional liability crisis could have a continuing negative impact on the cost of health care. Not only will the direct cost of professional liability coverage increase the cost of health care, but the indirect costs of defensive medicine also will continue to exert upward pressure on the costs of care. The increasing cost of professional liability insurance premiums also could have a negative effect on access to medical care in some geographic areas. For example, several localities have experienced a loss of obstetrical services as a result of rising professional liability premiums.

Theme 2. As cost containment pressures continue to grow, pressures will mount to develop effective methods for evaluating and assuring the quality of health care.

Methods of reimbursing physicians may alter traditional physician patient relationships. Current proposals to alter the way physicians are reimbursed under the Medicare program could impact on the quality of care delivered to Medicare patients.

The federal government can be expected to continue to intervene in the health care system. Some of this intervention will constitute increased interference in the practice of medicine. The need for organized medicine to represent the interests of physicians and patients is likely to increase.

Business and labor can be expected to continue to be concerned about the cost of care. Medical practice data may be scrutinized by groups that never before expressed interest in such information. New types of relationships are likely to develop between physicians and business/labor communities.

Third parties may attempt to overly influence how medicine is practiced through their reimbursement mechanisms. Third parties may also attempt to influence the setting in which certain medical services are delivered. Again, many of these activities will constitute increasing interference in the practice of medicine.

Theme 3. Advances in medical technology will continue to strongly influence the environment of medicine.

Changes in technology represent a most potent long range force for change in the environment of medicine. Advances in medical technology will provide physicians with more effective methods of diagnosis and treatment of disease. Advances will provide relief for many patients whose conditions would otherwise have been hopeless.

Technological innovations may be increasingly scrutinized from a cost-benefit standpoint by third party payers and others.

Changes in medical technology will continue to be a potent force in the growth of various specialties in medicine.

Theme 4. Fundamental shifts in the demographic characteristics of the US population will have a major effect on the long range demand for medical care services.

The changing demographic characteristics will place added emphasis on treating the medical conditions of the elderly population. Consequently, treatment of chronic conditions will gain added emphasis.

The shifting age composition of the population is likely to create shifts in the demand for physicians' services by specialty. For example, the number of births per year is likely to fall throughout the 1990s, which will have an impact on the demand for obstetric and pediatric care. The increasing numbers of elderly people, however, suggest that the demand is likely to grow for the services of Internists, Radiologists, General/ Family Practitioners, Neurologists, physicians specializing in chronic diseases, and other physicians who treat older patients.

The migration patterns of the US population suggest that the growth in demand for physicians' services is likely to vary substantially from area to area. In general, states in the South and West will experience rapid growth, while states in the Northeast and Midwest will experience a slower growth in demand.

The increase or decline in the prevalence of diseases will have an impact on the demand for physicians' services. AIDS, for example, will likely increase the demand for Internists, General/Family Practitioners, and other primary care providers.

Theme 5. The supply of physicians is projected to increase at a faster rate than the US population overall.

Young physicians should expect competition will increase during their practice careers. Remaining flexible with respect to areas of specialization, new skills, and practice location should assist young physicians in maintaining interesting and rewarding medical careers.

The increasing supply of physician manpower will, almost certainly, increase access to medical care, result in an improvement in the health status of the public, and allow physicians more time to spend with each patient.

As specialists continue to locate in nonmetropolitan areas and small cities, referral patterns for specialized care may change. Fewer patients from rural areas may be referred to major metropolitan hospitals for medical care. This change may be beneficial for those patients who will no longer have to travel long distances for medical care. However, specialists in metropolitan areas may begin to face more direct competition from their rural colleagues.

The growing supply of physicians and the shifting specialty composition are likely to raise concerns about the mechanisms that influence the specialty mix of physicians. Questions are likely to arise about the forces that link the future demand for physicians' services in a specialty with the availability of residency positions in that specialty.

Theme 6: Governmental initiatives are likely to continue to be a major source of change in the environment of medicine.

The combination of governmental concern over rising health care costs and governmental power to alter the health care financing and delivery systems through legislation and regulation could lead to substantial changes in the environment of medicine in the near future.

The federal government is likely to alter its method of reimbursing physicians under Medicare, which is likely to have ramifications for private third party reimbursement mechanisms.

Theme 7: Health policy issues will become increasingly politicized.

The debate of health care issues will continue to expand beyond the medical community. Many health policy issues may no longer be determined by sound medical practice, but by political factors.

Theme 8: Changes in the environment of medicine may lead to unexpected divisions and alliances on health policy issues.

The intensity of economic competition in the health sector is likely to continue to increase because of the increasing supply of health care personnel and because of the changes in the financing of care. Increased competition is likely to cause realignments among key participants in the health care sector, often depending upon the particular issue involved.

The pressure to contain health care expenditures is a fundamental force that is causing evolution in the roles of the major participants in the health sector. In general, the major participants have become more active in attempting to modify, to some degree, the health care system in order to restrain costs.

Theme 9: The environment of the health care sector will become more uncertain.

Given the number and magnitude of changes that have taken place over the past decade in the American health care system, as well as the current and projected environmental trends, it will become increasingly difficult to predict the shape of the health care system in the future.

As Medicine prepares to meet these challenges, it will face the over-arching issue of the nurture and protection of professionalism. This implies a strengthened commitment on the part of physicians to self-discipline and service to patients and to the public interest. Such a social contract will help assure independence in clinical decision-making and a strong patient-doctor relationship. The Council on Long Range Planning and Development believes that these elements of professionalism are the ground substance of high quality medical care at reasonable cost which is the goal of the American people.

Conclusion